A Not So Lonely Journey

CC Thompson
Walter Zerrenner

A Not So Lonely Journey
Compiled by CC Thompson and Walter Zerrenner
Published by Journey Publish LLC
Appleton, WI 54914
JourneyPublish@gmail.com

Copyright © 2021 by Journey Publish LLC
All rights reserved. No part of this book may be reproduced, stored in, or introduced into a retrieval system, or transmitted to any form, or by any means to include electronic, mechanical, photocopying, recording, or otherwise without the prior written permission of the individual authors.

This book should not be used as a substitute for the advice of medical or legal professionals.

First printing, March 2021
Printed in the United States of America
Library of Congress Control Number: 2020951287
ISBN: 978-1-7322069-2-2
ePUB ISBN: 978-1-7322069-3-9

Cover photo credit Webtech.com
10 9 8 7 6 5 4 3 2 1

DEDICATION

This book is dedicated to the amazing caregivers who have joined together to share their thoughts and journeys to support other caregivers and to help family, friends, co-workers, and employers better understand the journey of caring for a loved one.

SHARING THE JOURNEY

Disclaimer	i
Introduction	iii
A Love Note	1
And Then There Was Covid	5
Carolyn: The Girl I Married	11
Earning Perspective	29
Give Me Patience	51
Into the Fog	55
Lifesavers for Me	61
Living in the Moment	65
Love Survives the Journey	83
My Day as a Caregiver	95
Not Doing Enough	107
Now What	113
Our Journey	117
Our Life Puzzle	129
Reflections of a Caregiver	161
The Best and the Worst	171

The Other Talk	175
The Perfect Life	181
The Right Doctor	185
Treated Differently	189
Two Strangers in the House	195
What I Wish I Had Known	201
What is a Caregiver	205
Where Did the Laughter Go	209
Thank You	213
Afterword	215
About	217
Disclaimer	223

DISCLAIMER

These thoughts and journeys are written and shared by family caregivers in their own words, not by medical or legal professionals.

Any information shared in this book is not intended to be, nor should it be, interpreted as medical or legal advice.

Medical and legal questions or concerns should be directed to your medical and legal professionals.

A NOT SO LONELY JOURNEY

"May you find comfort and support on your journey."

INTRODUCTION

In 2018, family caregivers came together and created a book called *A Lonely Journey*. After the book was published, other family caregivers reached out asking for an opportunity to share in a second book. Caregivers often say the journey at first appears to be very lonely, but as they come together with other caregivers and share their knowledge and experiences, the road becomes *A Not So Lonely Journey*.

We applaud the family caregivers who, in their own words, shared their thoughts and journeys to make this second book possible. We have respected the privacy of those caregivers who have requested to remain anonymous.

The intent of this second book is to continue to support family caregivers as well as to help family, friends, co-workers and employers better understand the journey of a family caregiver.

As each submission is unique to itself, there are no numerated chapters. The submissions are arranged in alphabetical order based on their titles. The alphabetizing also allows the ability to flip through the book to easily refer to a favorite later.

It is our honor to give a voice to family caregivers. A special thank you to the Aline Zerrenner Dementia Friendly Fund for making this sharing possible.

A sincere appreciation and thank you to all family caregivers for your daily dedication to your loved ones. May you find comfort and support on your journey.

CC Thompson and Walter Zerrenner

"It is our honor to give a voice to family caregivers."
—CC and Walt

A NOT SO LONELY JOURNEY

"I choose to stay."

A LOVE NOTE

We have a good life. I have nothing to complain about or to look back on with tears. You are the love of my life. You are everything I could have hoped for and more. I put no blame on you for these past years of caring for you. We have had our share of difficult days, but we manage to continue to get through them and to start fresh the next morning.

I know, at this point, it is extremely difficult for you to express your feelings about me or about anything for that matter. At times, you show anger. I want you to know that I do not take your anger personally. I am just as frustrated and angry as you are at this disease which has taken so much from you. I simply hide it well when I am with you, so I can enjoy our time together.

Do not have pity for me or guilt for yourself. Out of love, I choose to stay with you and to care for you. I feel no obligation—just love. I know strongly in my heart that you would reciprocate for me.

I want you to know the twinkle that I see in your eyes, some days, fills my heart with joy. I feel your love when you squeeze my hand a little firmer than usual. I see love when I look at you.

Every day that we are together, we continue to build memories for ourselves and for others around us. Memories that will outlast us both.

Neither of us knows what the future holds, but know that you can count on my love now and always. We have a bond that cannot be broken by a disease. You may not be able to speak the words, but with your body language, I can still hear you say, "I love you."

—Love Always

A LOVE NOTE

"You can count on my love."

A NOT SO LONELY JOURNEY

"*Where did everyone go?*"

AND THEN THERE WAS COVID

Just like life, being a family caregiver has its ups and downs. I have learned isolation and loneliness are a part of the territory of being a family caregiver. I share this, not out of self-pity, but as reality.

We had a very active social life that included numerous longtime friends from college, high school, and even some from our childhoods. When it became obvious my husband was having some form of cognitive issues, I was amazed how quickly longtime friends took a step back. Actually, several steps back.

I was always the friend who stepped forward when one of our friends faced a hardship. Whether it was relationship issues, divorce, miscarriage, loss of a child, fire, loss of a job, or illness, etc., I was there for them. Where are those friends now for me?

In March 2020, Wisconsin went into a pandemic shutdown which I thought would only last two weeks. Family caregivers often feel isolated and alone, but the pandemic has only multiplied that feeling. Caregivers cannot take the chance of allowing others into their home, visiting others or even taking that much needed break of going to lunch with a friend. As of this writing, we are going into our tenth month of shutdown like the rest of the United States.

So far, I feel my husband and I have fared much better than I anticipated through this pandemic in many ways. Like others, we have been staying at home and wearing a mask when we absolutely need to leave the house. No one else has been in our vehicle or in our home.

Occasionally, our children and grandchildren will visit wearing masks in our driveway. Oh, how I long to cuddle my grandchildren and spend quality time with them like we used to. They have grown and changed so much in the last 10 months. How do we recover this lost time?

Through all of this, I have learned how to order groceries online which are delivered to our front door for a fee. To secure a weekly delivery spot, I set an alarm for 3:00 a.m. which, I have learned, is the time when the websites reset for their new available delivery dates. I have also learned I can fill my online shopping cart and have it ready for checkout when the new delivery dates are available. Yes, many times items have been out of stock, but not being able to get one of our favorite grocery items is nothing compared to what others are dealing with in this pandemic.

Doctor appointments have changed as well. Phone calls from doctors do not feel like adequate substitutes, but sometimes that is what is necessary to get a prescription refilled.

When possible, we go for car rides. It feels good

just to see other people whether they are in their vehicles or out walking. I need that reassurance of knowing we are not the only two people on the planet as it so often feels.

Now and then, I do try to reach out to old friends, but it feels they have moved on without us. The fact that they don't reach out back says a lot. I often wonder during this pandemic how busy can they be?

I am sharing this because I want to encourage everyone as a friend or family member to step up and let a family caregiver know that you care and appreciate what they do on a daily basis. Call them today. Send a note or email letting them know that you are thinking of them. Send them flowers or a small gift of appreciation. Your small act of kindness will go a long way in the life and support of a family caregiver.

—Anonymous

AND THEN THERE WAS COVID

"An act of kindness goes a long way."

A NOT SO LONELY JOURNEY

"A smile says so much."

CAROLYN: THE GIRL I MARRIED

As I began to write this in 2019 for my annual Christmas letter, I was feeling the consequences of being a 10 year dementia caregiver. I often think about the fact that our situation is never going to get better. My happiness now depends upon whether or not my wife, Carolyn, smiles or doesn't smile.

If she smiles when I first awaken her when she is sleeping in her chair, I know it is going to be a good day. If she doesn't smile, and has trouble getting up out of her chair, then I know it probably won't be such a good day.

My daily routine is focused on the best ways that I have found to interact with Carolyn. When you have someone who just sits all day long, or just stares into space, you want to find ways to communicate with them.

Two wise people, who work at the place where Carolyn now lives, noticed that I was talking about her like she wasn't there. I felt it was alright because I thought she wasn't aware of things. They pointed out although she can't verbalize, if I watch her eyes she will sometimes react to what is being said.

I am so appreciative they made me aware of this. Now I talk to her more like I used to years ago. Even though she doesn't answer, I have noticed that she probably understands more than I realized. She especially likes it when I talk about our children, grandchildren, her brothers and sisters, and when we dated.

Every day we would go for a stroll in the hallways where she now lives. Our walk includes going up and down 20 steps because I fear Carolyn is losing her mobility.

We visit with people along the way in the independent, assisted living, and in the memory care unit where Carolyn lives. The residents there are especially appreciative of any kindness shown towards them. Being able to help bring a smile to these residents really cheers me up.

I can sense others who have experienced, or are going through what I am experiencing, because they will give me a hug or other positive physical touches as they talk to Carolyn.

Even if she doesn't respond, those who have experience with dementia will keep trying to get her attention through touch and verbalization. Others don't say anything, and that is also okay. Before Carolyn had dementia, I didn't know what to do or say to someone with dementia either. Hopefully, this letter will help others to better understand and know what to do.

The ultimate activity for my spouse is music. I can honestly say music has really helped to retain what is left in our relationship.

We especially enjoy ballroom dancing and have

been taking dancing lessons for the past few years. Carolyn smiles more when we are dancing than any other activity. I love it!

With the progression of the disease, even dancing was becoming more difficult. Our turns and our steps were slower. However, she still has a bounce in her step when she hears music. I also believe dancing helps her balance. We will keep on dancing as long as she can.

Five years ago, Carolyn and I celebrated our 45th wedding anniversary and went on a second honeymoon. I am so glad I did not wait until our 50th. We have gone from walking around the block to taking a little stroll around her memory care unit.

At first, we lost basic conversation between us. However, we still had cute gestures like her smiles, dimples and her kiddingly sticking out her tongue at me.

Then I added her in my presentations that I do for nursing homes, schools, senior centers, memory cafes, etc. She became Mrs. Cat in the Hat, Mrs. Santa Claus, and even a donkey in one of my campfire presentations. It was great fun for both of us and, though her role was minor, she laughed a lot.

We met when I asked her to dance in 1968. As the Alzheimer's progressed, I realized how even though she could not carry on conversations anymore, we could still enjoy dancing. So, we took lessons whenever we could. Sadly, eventually she could not participate in dance classes or travel well anymore.

Problem Solving—I asked the dance instructor if she could come to Carolyn's memory care unit once a week for lessons. She agreed and was able to show me how to dance with Carolyn despite her limited mobility. Soon after, Carolyn became dependent on her wheelchair.

When I told the instructor I thought our dancing days were done, she surprised me again. She taught me how to dance around Carolyn's wheelchair. However, right after that, the pandemic restrictions took place.

Music makes Carolyn smile along with silly animal pictures, hugs, little children, and ice cream. If I had only known the power of ice cream when we were dating, I would have forgone the flowers and candy. Ha, ha.

How I Cope

Writing and presenting my thoughts seems to help me cope with Carolyn's dementia as well. I do occasionally break down emotionally, but that's okay because it just shows that I care. I feel it also helps others to better understand what it is like to be a caregiver in love.

By writing this, presenting various programs, and supporting the Alzheimer's and Dementia Alliance of Wisconsin (ADAW), I feel I am honoring Carolyn. Her plight has made me a better person. I now realize, more than ever, the importance of doing things with loved ones. As her caregiver, happiness is when I make her happy. As I say once again, I live for her smiles.

In several ways the Alliance (ADAW) has honored me this past year. They recommended me to be interviewed several times as a caregiver, and chose me as an honorary chairperson of the local Grant County Alzheimer's Walk. I was also part of a PowerPoint presentation on the theme of how Carolyn and I still have fun.

I feel I have a new mission in my life. With the publicity I received as an honorary Alzheimer's Walk chairperson, others have approached me saying they were emotionally moved.

As a caregiver, I can personalize the facts. They tell me their stories and ask where to go to get help. They often have been trying to keep it a secret or are realizing that they do need help as a caregiver, just as I did.

I tell other caregivers to contact the Adult

Disability Resource Center (ADRC) in their community and I give them a card on how to contact the Alzheimer's and Dementia Alliance of Wisconsin (ADAW). As I hand others the card, I look them in the eye and say, "It will change your life." The same reciprocal positive feelings I received through teaching sixth-graders, I now feel helping other caregivers on their journeys.

One of my most supportive groups is the wonderful fellows I met while at Loras College. We recently had our 50th class reunion. It was while at Loras that I strengthened my faith, chose my career, made wonderful friends, and during Easter vacation in 1968 met Carolyn. Those were my very good "good old days."

I stay active by ushering at church, reading, teaching a fourth grade religion class, amateur radio, Cat in the Hat programs, local history presentations, and leading indoor campfires. Recently, I even did my Elvis routine for a women's group. I also give presentations to local civic groups, schools, and elderly institutions about Alzheimer's.

I suppose I am bragging, but these things help me feel good inside and help me to forget Carolyn's plight. She used to sing Jingle Bells with me as Mrs. Santa Claus and would accompany me as Mrs. Cat in the Hat. However, doing these things are too difficult for her now.

Adjusting to her life changes is not easy and causes me some emotional strain each time a new problem develops. A caregiver becomes a constant problem solver as the disease evolves and your loved one's condition continues to deteriorate.

You can do more than you think you can. You can make a difference, especially if you are doing it to help others and not just yourself. Do things for both others and yourself and you will have those internal good vibrations that will make your life more enjoyable.

Family and friends are a great support to both

of us. I have found that if I ask, people will help. This helps me cope as a dementia caregiver.

We celebrated our 50th wedding anniversary on May 30, 2020. As I now reflect on my marriage of 50 years, I realize Carolyn had Alzheimer's dementia for at least 12 of those 50 years. She is now in the final stages of this disease. I have concluded that the most difficult issue has been how this disease has slowly taken away the intimacy we had which is so important to a successful marriage. Friends, family, and support groups are helpful, but they cannot replace the intimacy that you share with your spouse. Without intimacy, there is loneliness.

Besides the word "intimacy," other important words are "problem solving" and "don't wait." Don't wait to get help. Time is important with dementia. You want to do things while your loved one can still help with decisions and still enjoy activities.

When I first knew of Carolyn's dementia, I will

never forget what a college professor told me. His wife had just passed away. He turned to me and said, "I am very sorry to hear that. I feel sorry for you." People's sympathy sure helps, but it cannot solve a problem like this by itself.

Then there is the guilt that has now, for the first time, entered into the picture. You might ask why I would have guilt feelings. Haven't you done everything possible? Yes, but now with Carolyn in the final stages, I feel guilty because I find myself just wishing it was all over and done with.

I would rather wish for a cure, but I know that is not going to happen. I was helped immensely about these feelings when a priest on TV was speaking about Alzheimer's caregivers, like myself. He said we should not feel guilty about such thoughts.

Another very nice lady from a support group I attend, who lost her spouse, scolded me for mentioning guilt. She also loved her spouse dearly, but both of their lives were being wrecked by the disease. Now with his passing, she is able to once again get her life back together.

Carolyn and I have been on a long journey for the past 12 or more years. It has not been an easy one. I was doing okay as long as I could get her to smile. We could go for walks and most of all dance. I knew we needed those three things so badly in our lives.

All the other terrible things that happen to other people with Alzheimer's were now happening to us. Around the end of March, the final stages of this disease set in very quickly. Suddenly, while we were doing our daily three dances in her room, she went down very quickly. Just as others had told me would happen, she could no longer push herself up even with my help. I knew then that she would now have to go to a different facility for more care.

At the new facility, Carolyn is now living out the final stages of dementia. She now requires a wheel chair, no longer smiles, and speaks mostly in gibberish while living in some kind of a hallucination world.

As if that is not bad enough, now with the pandemic, I can only see her through her window. I actually think it frightens her when she sees a man (me) looking at her through the window. The last positive memory I have is of us holding hands and listening to music.

At the previous facility, when we could still interact through dancing, walking, and smiles, I would visit daily for an hour. I so enjoyed our visits. However, now that she is in a different state of life and with the pandemic, I only go every couple of days and look into her window. I go less now because it is too emotional for me when I do visit.

I have many good friends and loving family who support me and care about me and yet I still feel the loneliest that I have ever felt. I can't blame anyone. It is just part of the process one naturally goes through when you lose a spouse. The difference is that with Alzheimer's dementia you have lost that person mentally and emotionally, but they are still physically here. They are now unable to show you the love you need that through God's gift holds a couple together. I long for her love again. Even though I realize that she is no longer capable of this, it does not make it any easier.

Nancy Reagan has referred to dementia as "the slow death." For more than 12 years I have seen Alzheimer's continually try to destroy our life together. Now with the pandemic, I am not even able to hold her hand. Carolyn is unable to comprehend who I am or what is going on when she is looking at me through a window.

I am especially thankful to several priests. They have been extremely helpful by being good listeners and reminding me to seek peace through prayer, and that time eventually helps to heal mental anguish. Emotions are strong and often hard to control. So many people have helped me to continue to be optimistic that my situation will make me a better person. I also get comfort from helping others who are now beginning this terrible journey with their spouse, parent, sibling, etc.

I had been feeling sorry for myself and tried not to think about her. For the first time, I felt I deserved a better life. I was feeling selfish. I missed Carolyn's companionship and intimacy so much. Thank goodness for the support of my friends and family who have been so kind.

Even when I was feeling guilty as a caregiver, many reminded me how much I loved Carolyn and how, only recently, was I not able to enjoy her companionship of dancing and intimacy through her smile.

While on one of my recent walks, I was thinking what can I do to get Carolyn back into my life. For a while, all I could think of were negative things. Then I thought, let's problem solve. That is when I decided to write family members asking them to write me about their fond memories of Carolyn. Once again, it was fun remembering the good times with Carolyn instead of thinking about the negative things. I got out old pictures and watched some old videos and listened to a lot of music from the good old days. Now I am putting together a booklet on all of our fondest memories of Carolyn. The children have some great memories of the simplest things.

As of this writing, it has been over nine months since I last held Carolyn's hand. On the last day before pandemic restrictions we held hands and listened to three songs we used to dance to everyday in her room: foxtrot, swing step, and a waltz.

Finally, there are two treasured private thoughts I'll share with you. The first is that I can't listen to Bobby Goldsboro's song "Honey" without a tear in my eye. That was Carolyn.

The second thought happened about a year ago when we were dancing a slow dance in our living room. Carolyn squeezed me like she used to when we were dating. That is such a small, but powerful memory. I will always treasure that moment and that memory.

—*Kent Scheuerell* ©2020

*"Finding perspective makes
the journey easier."*

EARNING PERSPECTIVE

In May of 2013, my mom fell face first onto a concrete sidewalk. She was 82. It was Mother's Day. She broke her left wrist in two places. She is left handed. She also broke her right foot. My second brother, who was in town, took her to the emergency room himself. She would never be the same again. The spiral into dementia began that day. Her doctor would tell me that traumatic injuries can initiate a decline.

Had I known that the day before this fall would be the last day I would ever see her "normal," I may have paid closer attention to what we were doing. I might have tried to remember more details. I would probably have taken some pictures.

But the Dementia Monster is a cunning villian.

It does not warn you when it is about to strike. It doesn't follow any rules or play fair. It sneaks up and sucker punches you just when you thought you had it figured out. Dementia takes a little bit of its victim every week. A memory today, some hair tomorrow, and next week maybe a tooth.

After the fall that day, my mom would never be normal again. It was literally that fast. She changed in one day—overnight. The Dementia Monster had arrived. I would spend years saying hello to my new mom as I grieved the loss of my old mom. The perspectives I would gain would be earned the hard way—six years later with the five stages of grief.

May 2019, Mom is 88 now. She has caregivers every day, twice a day. They've been coming for four years now. My mom doesn't have Alzheimer's disease. She has a different form of dementia. On her birthday a few weeks earlier, just she and I had a little party to celebrate. I brought flowers and gave her some new puzzles, a new hair brush and some scrunchies for her long hair. We ate chocolate cupcakes.

My second brother and his wife called long distance and sang Happy Birthday on the phone. My first brother sent fancy chocolates and two miniature rose bushes to plant in her tiny yard.

The caregiver that day used her own cell phone to take a photo of mom, and then, using one of the fun filters, added glowing birthday candles to mom's image. I made a list for mom of some famous people that she was still younger than such as: Betty White, Dick Van Dyke, Kirk Douglas, Olivia de Havilland. All of them were still living at the time. My mom was still a whippersnapper compared to them.

I don't know if she remembered anything about her birthday celebration that day. It may have flitted away before I even got home. When she called me at five that evening, as she has done every night for a couple decades, I did not ask and she did not bring it up.

It has been six years since my mom nosedived into dementia with that terrible fall. She's still in her mobile home, living by herself, with caregivers and hot meal deliveries every day. She is more frail, but still feisty. More confused, but still grounded.

My mom has become old. Every year that goes by, I think she can't get any "older." Her thin white hair, her halting walk, and her brown cataracts all testify to her age. Her face is deeply lined showing where every smile has been. Her hunched over posture betrays her intent to appear strong. I keep thinking that THIS is the "oldest" she will get. But every year, she grows weaker, frailer. More hair falls away. More memories leave her forever. She gets older.

But as old as she gets, her inner self is always there. Even as my mom advances further into the recesses of her past, there are parts of her that are not lost. Her soul is still there. The mantras of her life are still there. "I can do it myself." "Be nice to others." "Smile." Her emotional matrix is still intact. Amen.

The main thing I notice about this six year mark is a personal milestone for myself. I've stopped grieving daily for my lost mother. I don't mean that I don't have my bouts of anger or disappointment. My perceived lack of knowing "what to do next" is still an impetus for profound despair. I still cry and even wail at the unfairness of it all.

The actual grieving has stopped. There may be a big hole to get over when the time comes that I lose her completely and forever; but sometimes when someone has spent years watching a loved one decline, all the grieving is done by the time the end comes. I have said goodbye to my old mom. Will I need to say another one when I lose my "new" mom?

It has taken six years, but I think the grieving

has ended. Is the long hello over? Or have I just developed a crust? I don't know. It feels like it has ended. I've been through all the stages—denial, anger, bargaining, depression, and acceptance. I see it clearly now.

Denial—At first, it was very challenging to think my mom may never be "normal" anymore. I would think, "Maybe this is just temporary. Maybe she'll get better when her broken bones heal." I didn't want to think that the mom I knew was gone. The reality was unfaceable. I spent the first full year in denial.

Anger—I was filled with consuming anger. Anger at the Dementia Monster. Anger at my own incompetence. Anger at everyone in the world who didn't have to deal with this. Anger at my brothers, who lived a thousand miles away, because I felt abandoned. I remember even being angry at a sweet middle aged librarian when I asked for a book to be reserved for me—a book about Alzheimer's disease.

She didn't know how to spell "Alzheimer's" and I had to spell it for her as if she had never heard of it before. How did SHE get to avoid this hell while I had to navigate it every day?

I told God every day that I hated him for leaving the Dementia Monster on my doorstep. I screamed, "Why don't you FIX this?! How can you be so cruel?!" Even my parents' bitter divorce 45 years prior hadn't angered me as much as thinking God had forsaken me. A cheating boyfriend in my teens hadn't riled me as much.

Bargaining—I thought if I became a better daughter, then maybe my mom would be "normal" again.

Depression—Oh boy, the two depressions I went through were debilitating. I cried on the bathroom floor. On the front porch. On the couch. I lost weight. Gained weight. Slept too much or didn't sleep at all. I would fight my depressions by sometimes taking long walks. I've exercised for years by walking.

Sometimes I would go to one of my long trails and say to myself, "I'm just going to walk until all I can think about is how tired and sore I am." I would put on a knapsack for added burden.

And finally, Acceptance—Lately, there is a weird calm amid what is still a difficult storm. This has become more a familiar chore than an overwhelming mantle. More like milking a cow every day than corralling a daily stampede. More like hoeing the garden every day than battling a daily hailstorm. Acceptance is relief. But it can't be faked.

The five stages of grief, except for the last one, are a sore path. All of them are in my back pocket now as evidence. Explanations of why I have so many emotional bruises. All endured with pain and angst. Not wrapped in pretty packages, but in plain brown paper.

Adversity is like a gauntlet. A gauntlet is two tight lines of people, shoulder to shoulder, facing each other. Then you are forced to run down between the two lines of people as fast as you can, getting hit and punched by everyone in the lines as you run past them. There is no shortcut. The only way out is straight through. As fast as you can. The grief gauntlet has taken me six years to run through.

This revelation that the grieving seemed to have stopped came over me quickly in just one day. I had stopped thinking that mom would get better. I was proficient now at entering her world and understanding her new limitations.

I HAVE done a bang-up job of getting her this far. I HAVE been a good daughter and every year that my mom lives longer is evidence of that. I started feeling better about myself. I had stopped beating myself up for perceived failings and started appreciating myself. I noticed that I felt lighter. Mom's dementia was not my fault. The paradigm had shifted.

I had another revelation. It was now summer of 2019. I still had not told my mom about the death of my father, her ex-husband, a year earlier. I had planned to keep it from her for the rest of her life. I didn't want to have to keep telling her over and over again, so I just didn't tell her at all.

I was still answering all her questions about him with as truthful a lie as I could muster: "Have you seen your father lately?" "No, not lately." "Do you play Scrabble with your father?" "No." "How is he doing?" "I don't know. I'll find out." "Is he okay?" "He was the last time I talked to him."

But it was a difficult summer for other reasons. I was overwhelmed with "mom-emergencies." They came one on top of another. I grew to hate the idea of an "emergency." The word started to lose its meaning. When you have one emergency right after another, are they really emergencies anymore, or are they now normalcy?

First, a pressure sore developed on her bottom

and had to be treated. It involved two unplanned doctor appointments and additional caregiver visits.

Then directly right on the heels of that, she had an abrupt decline. It was like falling off a cliff again. Just like the very first day after her fall six years before when we were all agape at the sudden change.

This time, in the summer of 2019, the sudden change was just as alarming. In my view, she declined 60% in three days. She did not know what day, time, or season it was. She confabulated outrageous stories when we talked each evening on the phone for the nightly check-in. Confabulations are stories, conjured and imagined, that the dementia patient believes to be true, but are not.

One story was about a strange man entering her mobile home without knocking and then calmly leaving when he saw her. Each time she told me this story, over the course of five minutes, details would change. First she was in her bedroom, and then she was on her couch. First it was daytime when this happened, then it was nighttime. I asked only one question, "What did he look like?" She couldn't answer. I was forced to file a police report even though I had no details to give them. What if it really happened?

Another confabulation was about how she was now living "downtown." She would tell me, "I'm downtown! They put me in a brand new mobile home right next to where I work. Didn't they tell you? I live downtown now. Right next to the Farmer's Market on Wednesdays. You know the Farmer's Market? Right next to where I work. Didn't they tell you?"

I freaked out. I said that one thing you're never supposed to say to someone with dementia, "Mom, what are you talking about? You're not making any sense." Was this it? Had her time come?

More emergency doctor visits. "We must see her

now, to make sure she doesn't have a UTI. TODAY! This is an EMERGENCY!" Did they not know I'm just one person? That I was running out of steam? Run, run, run. Now!

I fell to pieces in the doctor's office, sobbing uncontrollably. I couldn't talk or answer any questions. I had to excuse myself and go to a secluded hallway to sob in private. They called a counselor in to come talk to me. A doctor appointment for my mom, to make sure she wasn't dying, had become all about ME.

It turned out that she did not have a UTI. She returned to her baseline. It was decided that this particular instance was an anomaly. Perhaps it was a micro TIA (Trans Ischemic Attack.) TIAs are mini strokes. Micro TIAs are mini mini strokes. Perhaps it was the result of dehydration. They didn't know.

Then without any time to catch my breath after that, there came two mobile home maintenance issues which turned into, yeah, EMERGENCIES! I crashed again. I melted down. I screamed and made tirades. Make it stop! Then I started to wonder. Could some of my frustration be self-induced? I thought about how some of my own shortcomings may be playing a hand in how I responded to these unexpected incidents.

Why did I feel like I was failing? Why was I so upset that I couldn't make everything fine with a swipe of my hand so that I could just relax? I just wanted to relax. Why was I so pissed off? I started thinking hard about my expectations not only about my mom, but also about myself.

At the time I was exhibiting at art fairs for a living. I remember, before all this dementia stuff started, I was preparing applications for the art fairs I wanted to be in that year.

Many people may not know that when you are an exhibitor at a fancy-pants art fair, you have to submit an application months in advance. You don't just show up the day of the show and set up.

Oh, no. You have to send photos of your work and your booth way ahead of time. And they better be outstanding, professional studio photos. You also have to fill out lengthy applications explaining why you think you should be accepted. You have to send your booth fees and jury (entry) fees in at the same time.

It's not free to set up a booth at an art fair. Some of them cost hundreds of dollars. The jury fee is so the organizers can hire professional judges to look over your photos and determine if you are good enough to be in their show. If you are not accepted, you get the booth fee back, but not the jury fee. Having to pay to be rejected is a punch in the gut.

One day, I was working on three applications whose deadlines were coming up. I had spread out everything on the kitchen table trying to keep my piles organized. I was closely examining all my photos and materials. I had picked up a photo and was holding it up to my face, inches away, looking at it through a loupe for flaws. My husband came in and saw me. He chuckled at the sight of me holding a photo inches from my face. I exclaimed, without looking up, "It has to be PERFECT!"

He laughed at me even louder. He mimicked me by holding a blank piece of paper up to his face and repeating my edict through comically gritted teeth, "IT HAS TO BE PERRRR-FECT!" as he shook the paper in the air. We both started laughing. We laughed long and hard until we could barely breathe. It's still a running joke between us.

I've always wanted to be perfect. I want everything I do to be perfect. I want to control everyone else so that they too can do perfect things in a perfect way. I rarely trust other people to do things as perfectly as I.

Most of the time, I have to accept the imperfections of life. Many times I choose to just do something myself so it is perfect. Then I grumble the whole time because, "I CAN'T DO EVERYTHING!

Geez, can't anyone else do anything?" Yes, it's a curse, being so perfect. I realized that I was letting this perfection imperfection of mine seep into my caring for my mom.

During that summer of 2019, my mom needed a new window air conditioner—right away! It was going to be 90 degrees soon and the old air conditioner didn't work anymore! Yes – yet another crisis that summer, number seven, I believe.

When my husband offered to put it in for her—for me—I recoiled. Good heavens no! That had to be done professionally. I would have to drop everything, drive all the way up there after meticulously coordinating times with an electrician so I could meet them there and pay them immediately. I was sure I was the only one who could do it the right way.

My husband, who has maintained our income properties for decades, reminded me that he knew how to put in a window air conditioner. I still resisted. I didn't want to admit that I wasn't perfectly up to getting this done myself. I wanted to be the admired one. The one who always does things perfectly. Gaze upon me, the good daughter.

But I was pooped. I was falling apart after this recent slew of "emergencies." They had come too fast on top of each other. I had not an ounce of reserve in me to give to my mom. I needed my husband's help. His offer to do it was exactly what I needed—a lifeline. I had to relent and just let him do it his way.

I surrendered my desire to be perfect so I could be whole again. I didn't micromanage my husband on this task. He drove to Mom's, put the air conditioner in, and did some caulking. I stayed home and worried the whole time that he would slip off the ladder, smash his head, be taken to the emergency room, be admitted to the hospital and never come home. All because I did not do it myself. Then I would spend the rest of my life blaming my mother. He was back home in a couple hours.

My unreasonable need to always be perfect was affecting how I took care of my mom. That was on me, not her. I can't be bitching about how no one helps me take care of her and then refuse the help when it comes just so I can bitch about how no one helps me. Wow. That's a mouthful. But there it is.

I didn't like learning this about myself. I didn't like having to admit to myself how imperfect I was. I always thought it was totally possible to be perfect and that if you weren't, you just weren't trying hard enough.

I didn't like seeing this person in the mirror. I didn't like realizing that I could be that manipulative. But it sure helped knowing all this. I didn't need to be perfect after all. Would this revelation change how I would go through this journey? Yes.

Later on, in that summer of never-ending EMERGENCIES!, I put into practice what I had learned about myself. This time, when yet another mom crisis emerged, I was busy taking care of a pretty big crisis of my own with my husband's hospitalization. I called my second brother, who was in town for summer hiatus. I asked him for help dealing with our mother's newest crisis and he helped. Boy, it was nice to not be afraid to be imperfect.

We all have imperfections. Sometimes we don't admit them and sometimes we simply can't see them. One of mine was thinking that I could accuse others of not being perfect, while pretending that I was.

Learning this one thing about myself wasn't easy. Like most revelations, it came suddenly in one day. There is a paradox in knowing that I am imperfect will not make me perfect. Just like being uncool does not make you ironically cool. I still wish it was possible to be perfect. It isn't.

Today, December 2020, my mom is almost 90.

She still lives in her mobile home that she bought all by herself decades ago. She has caregivers coming in every day, two to three times a day. A hot meal is delivered every evening because I had her gas stove disconnected years ago. She can't play her piano anymore, so I play for her and we sing together. Singing is how she communicates now. She smiles non-stop and somehow gets from one day to the next. It's clear to me now that when I do lose her forever, I will indeed grieve the loss of my new mom.

When this all started, I was afraid all laughter would now be fake, all news would be bad, and all outlooks would be grim. I was sure the sun would dim, the rains would come, and fudge would forever taste bitter. None of this actually happened. There is still real laughter between my mom and me. All news is not bad and fudge is still delicious. I earned these perspectives.

—Julie ©2020

"Caregiving requires patience."

GIVE ME PATIENCE

I had always thought of myself as a very patient person. I had no idea how much patience I was going to need when I began caring for my husband. Becoming a family caregiver gave patience a whole new meaning.

When I look at my husband, I see a full-grown man. His actions and words, however, do not match his physical appearance. Because my eyes and mind do not see a child, I get frustrated when he does not respond as an adult.

Personal hygiene can be a challenge which is not something I would expect from an adult, especially someone who was very aware of their personal hygiene previously. Showering or even getting him to change clothes can be quite the challenge some days.

Grocery shopping in particular can be quite the adventure. When possible, I go alone, but often I have to bring him with me. He loads the cart with cookies and sweets, which I would unload when he is not looking. My apologies to the staff that have to put the items back correctly.

For some reason, he feels he has to talk loudly in the stores and make our existence known. It has been suggested to me to have cards that I can hand out to people that state my husband has a cognitive condition. I do not feel comfortable with that suggestion and I just simply smile back when people look at us. Hopefully people can still see my smile behind my mask.

I would say my grandmother was the most patient person I have known. I often think about the great example she was and try to be like her. Patient, kind and good.

I was once told, "Pray for patience and God will

GIVE ME PATIENCE

give you challenges to improve your patience." That does make sense when you think about it. Being a spousal caregiver does challenge your patience, but love somehow seems to rise above what I lack in patience and gives me strength to get through another day.

—Praying For Patience

A NOT SO LONELY JOURNEY

"No one prepares you."

INTO THE FOG

I wanted there to be more. I wanted there to be a greater space between what he knew and what he did not. I wanted him to know less. To not understand.

No one prepares you for the awareness that they do not know. Awareness within themselves that they should know, but do not. I thought there would be more not knowing. A simple transition from knowledge to fog. Frustration builds because the awareness lingers longer than we hoped. Sorrow builds from seeing the look of despair on the faces of those asking the questions to which he should know the answers.

Pain is reflected as the fog builds between the answers he no longer can find and the reality that he knows they are there, but are now lost in the fog. It becomes a delicate dance with the fog. I have read everything I could get my hands on about the progression. I know the steps. I know the stages. I know how the fog will creep in and then actually creep out before creeping in even further to stay.

The fog doesn't know we need more time. It doesn't care that it takes so much and yet leaves even more in ruins in its path. The fog has no remorse and keeps on creeping, relentless.

Some days the visits are upbeat and lively. Conversation will occur and interaction will be sincere and real. Some days the visits are dark and lonely. There is no energy and it is solemn. Conversations do not come and interaction is forced and confused. A journey of moments. Increments of time ticking away in memories lost and facts forgotten. More and more succumbing to the fog.

And then, one day, I arrive for a visit. I am hopeful, cautiously hopeful. Maybe it will be

INTO THE FOG

a good day. Maybe there will be energy and conversations. Perhaps today the fog will be held at bay for just enough time to spare more sorrow.

The moment of truth. His room door opens. I hold my head high and I breeze in while ignoring the hovering fog. Its threatening presence choking the room. I walk my paces, I take my breath and I express myself with the greeting I bring.

And there it is. Like a strike from a ghost into my chest. Like the surface of water suddenly overtaking me. The light fading, pulling me to its depths, no matter how hard I swim. My breath is held for that moment.

My brain can barely take it in. I hear myself talking right over it. Smiling and carrying the conversation on in the room. My own voice echoing in my head. Motions are robotic. There is no feeling behind them.

I am now outside myself. I am watching how I maneuver the room. I am calm. I am collected. Yet in spite of my outer control, I can hear the screams in my head. I can feel my heart pounding out of my chest. I can feel myself pushing, wanting to run as fast as I can as far away as I can. I am shocked that I am actually still there patiently talking. It feels like torture.

There are not enough words in the world to describe this feeling. This moment. I am there. I am aware of the reality that has brought me to this second in time. And yet, there is nothing, nothing in this earthly existence that can prepare you for such a moment.

The weight of the situation is almost unbearable. I become aware of every sound. I feel every breath as if it is the most difficult thing I have ever had to do. The time eventually passes and I watch myself finish my visit. I am finally able to escape the requirement.

I am alone. My body begins to let go. My walls start to weaken. My knees weaken right along with them. From deep within there begins a tremble that comes to the surface and brings with it the tears that are so often kept in check. My body realizes what has happened before my brain can accept it. I shake and I cry and I begin to understand what my body is trying to say.

I feel it in my bones. I hear the words forming in my mind. I try with all my might to hold them back. To refuse the reality. To ignore the facts. But like water on a rampage it cannot be restrained. It cannot be stopped. The words that will break me into a million pieces. The words that I cannot take back. The words that leave me breathless. The words that my heart fights to hide from my mind. Finally I hear them. The words I knew would one day come.

My father does not remember me. I have slipped into the fog.

—Kelley L King ©2020

"Love is patient. Love is kind."

LIFESAVERS FOR ME

I won't sugar coat it. Being a family caregiver is tough. Love has to be stronger than the disease. There are times that I wondered if I can do another day, but I do. Love endured again.

These following verses from I Corinthians are a few of my favorites. I feel these reminders help me to be a better caregiver for my husband.

>*Love is patient.*
>
>*Love is kind.*
>
>*It does not envy.*
>
>*It does not boast.*
>
>*It is not proud.*
>
>*It does not dishonor others.*
>
>*It is not self-seeking.*
>
>*It is not easily angered.*

It keeps no record of wrongs.

Love does not delight in evil,

But rejoices with the truth.

It always protects,

Always trusts,

Always hopes,

Always perseveres.

Love never fails.

I have found support groups to be a tremendous outlet for me. The term "support group" sounds outdated. I think there is still a stigma attached to the words "support group," so caregivers shy away.

Needing to share and talk about your struggles is nothing any person should be ashamed of. Personally, I would prefer "Friendship Group" or "Coffee Group" or "Caregivers' Group" or "Lifesaver Group." The latter is what the group has been for me. A lifesaver! Does the group really need to even have a label?

LIFESAVERS FOR ME

If you have not found a group yet, I recommend that you at least give it a try. It's not all gloom and doom. If it is, then you need to find a new group. There is laughter in caregiving. There is comfort in not feeling alone. Strength comes in sharing.

Every human being needs "me time" and no one, especially caregivers, should ever feel guilty about needing some time for themselves. "Me time" refreshes the body, soul, and mind. Take care of you, so you have what you need to adequately take care of your loved one. On an airplane you are told to put on your own oxygen first, then help your loved ones. That applies here as well. Take care of your emotional wellbeing.

Are you due for some "me time?" Resources for respite care are available through your county ADRC office or at RespiteCareWi.org. Do not put "me time" off as your own life and your loved ones depend on your wellbeing.

—Sam ©2020

"Our new normal"

LIVING IN THE MOMENT

Aline Mary Hirner was born July 29, 1941, in Edison, New Jersey, to Mary and Robert Hirner. She was their only child.

After graduating from Perth Amboy High School, Aline attended Montclair College. She graduated from Montclair with a Bachelor of Arts in Education. In the fall of 1963, she accepted a position as a math teacher. We met in the summer of 1964.

I was born July 8, 1941, in New York City as the oldest of five children. After graduating from high school, I enlisted in the Marines. I was honorably discharged from the Marine Corps, in July 1963, after serving four years and reaching the rank of Corporal.

Taking advantage of the G.I. Bill, I enrolled in college and attended night school while I worked full time.

During the summer of 1964, Aline and I met on the beach in Bayhead, New Jersey. We hit it off, married a year later, and built a life together. We have two children and five grandchildren. I retired in 2005, and we moved to Wisconsin to be with our daughter and four grandchildren. If we had opted for the Sunbelt, which was a consideration, we would not have been able to travel to see the grandchildren.

Our move to Wisconsin proved to be most rewarding for the two oldest grandsons. The boys were from our daughter's first marriage and were living in a split custody situation. We played an important role in the grandson's lives and helped to shape their future. That would have not been possible if we had retired anywhere else.

It would have been a travesty if Aline had not

been part of their lives and watch them grow into fine young men. She would later forget those days, but the boys did not, nor did I. The boys were so patient and understanding with her memory lapses. It was heartwarming. They would answer her repetitive questions as if it were the first time she asked, and it was for her.

The Early Progression

It was during our annual vacation in New York City in December 2006, when I noticed the first signs that something was wrong. We spent a week in New Jersey visiting friends and family.

The second week we were in New York City staying in mid-town Manhattan. We dined at Smith & Wolenskys the first evening and the following morning Aline did not feel well. She was very tired and wanted to remain in bed. She slept in until 11:00 a.m. and then we ate brunch in the hotel coffee shop.

After brunch, Aline said she was still tired and she went back to bed. That evening, we had room service and afterward she slept some more. I hoped it was a matter of the trip and excitement getting to her and that she would feel better the next day.

She slept in again and we ate in the hotel coffee shop again. The pattern continued for the next couple of days and she had no interest in doing anything that we had planned. There was something very wrong.

This was a woman who loved New York, particularly during the holiday season. Normally we would be walking all around the city, taking in the store front windows, Rockefeller Center with the Christmas Tree, Radio City Music Hall Christmas show, dining at our favorite restaurants and greeting the owners who we knew personally. That was the Aline I knew. Not this person who didn't want to do anything but sleep.

We cut the trip short and returned home

to Wisconsin. Our family physician listened to my recount of the trip and her behavior. He recommended an MRI and to have it interpreted by a psychiatrist. The test was scheduled before we left his office.

The MRI was performed and the interpretation made by a neuropsychologist. The diagnosis was Mild Cognitive Impairment (MCI). Looking at the MRI, there was white matter on the brain, evidence of a mini-stroke.

Thinking back before the New York trip, I had noticed some changes in Aline's forgetfulness. I had just attributed that to our aging process.

In 2007, we were still members at a country club and enjoyed playing golf. One day after ladies' golf, Aline arrived home 45 minutes later than expected. It was only a 10-minute drive from the country club. She had no explanation as to why it took so long, nor could she recall the route she took home. It frightened her to have that memory lapse, and at that moment, we agreed that she shouldn't drive.

Her memory continued to get worse, and I noticed it was getting more difficult to leave her home alone for longer periods of time.

I had to shut down my consulting business, as I could not travel and take her to an unfamiliar city. I just landed a very lucrative consulting engagement with a large healthcare system, and I had to turn it down.

The neuropsychological tests were administered by a psychiatrist in 2007 and then again in 2008. There was no significant decline indicated with the two tests. However, a second MRI showed the presence of more mini strokes, but none as severe as the first stroke. The diagnosis was changed to Vascular Dementia.

We had to make some significant lifestyle changes including vacation plans. We had a three week trip to Italy planned which I canceled. The big concern about traveling, especially out of the country, was what would she do if something happened to me.

There were still plenty of fun things to do. We took trips to Ski Brule and the Wisconsin Dells with the family. We were season ticket holders and Annual Partners at the Fox Cities Performing Arts Center. Aline loved to dine out, and we ate at our favorite Italian restaurant two or three times a week.

Grandchildren were involved in a number of activities which we always attended. We accepted the things that we could not do any longer, but enjoyed the things we still could. That is still true today. We call it "Living in the Moment."

Cooking, cleaning, medication management, and driving to medical appointments became my new normal. Dementia wasn't the fairytale retirement we had planned, but I was determined to focus on what we still could do together, and how I could make a difference.

We started participating in Memory Cafés through the Fox Valley Memory Project. In fact, we were part of the very first Memory Café. Aline continued playing bridge with her friends, and we took daily tours of our yard to look at the flowers and trees.

Early Onset of Alzheimer's

In March of 2009, additional neuropsychology testing revealed that Aline had moved into the early stage of Alzheimer's. The psychiatrist told us that we did not need to come to appointments anymore and suggested that we start looking at resources. She handed me a stack of information about Alzheimer's, along with a suggested reading list. I was advised to contact a neurologist for Aline's continuum of care.

Knowing the day would come when I could no longer care for Aline at home, we evaluated the memory care facilities in the Fox Valley. We visited and toured many of them and ranked them based on Aline's comfort level.

I began my education about Alzheimer's in 2009 using the information provided by the psychiatrist. I read a number of books and white papers, and I looked at online resources. Much of the information helped me understand the current situation and prepare for the days ahead.

I was still active, playing in a golf league, skiing, and working out at the Y. Aline was now at the stage where it was difficult to leave her home alone. At first, I would work out at the Y and be home by 8:00 a.m. before she was awake. Even if she was up, she would see the schedule on the whiteboard. That all changed when she forgot to read the whiteboard and panicked if I wasn't home.

An in-home care organization was referred to me, and I looked into their services. It worked out perfectly as all the caregivers were excellent, and

Aline liked all of them. A couple of them even became her friends.

We had purchased long-term care insurance in 2001, never expecting to use it so soon or for Alzheimer's. The in-home care organization was an approved agency and there was no problem being reimbursed for their services.

Being home alone with Aline was still challenging, dealing with the redundant questions and occasional hallucinations. Having a caregiver in the house to give me time away was also very important for my own health. Using in-home care services allowed me to keep Aline at home for as long as possible.

On December 1, 2014, Aline moved to a memory care neighborhood, which is a specialized community that can be free-standing or part of a care facility for seniors diagnosed with dementia, memory loss, or Alzheimer's. We had reached the point where I was stressed out and not sleeping

LIVING IN THE MOMENT

well, and my own health was at risk. Aline had become very clingy and did not want me to even leave the room. She was hallucinating at night and causing me to have sleepless nights. It was time.

Aline adjusted very well at the memory care neighborhood. Her neurologist said it was because we did not wait too long to make the transition. I continued to take her out to shows, to her favorite restaurants, and to family activities. We kept a balance in her life, recognizing that I could not do the things that the care facility could do, but I also did the things that the facility could not. During this time, I became very active with volunteer work. Staying active helps me deal with my own loneliness.

In May 2019, Aline had another mini-stroke and fell and broke her left hip. She had hip replacement surgery and had to be moved to another facility for a month of rehabilitation and physical therapy.

Then on Labor Day, Aline fell and broke her right

hip. Once again, it was hip replacement surgery, rehabilitation, and physical therapy. This time I made the decision to keep Aline's move permanent at the facility that also provided rehab services.

These days, we are working on Aline's mobility in hopes that I can start taking her out in the warmer weather. She is pretty much confined to the wheelchair, but we are using the walker on a limited basis.

I visit Aline at least every other day. It is becoming more difficult to visit as she always thinks that I am there to take her home. Her short-term memory is very poor, and she asks the same questions repeatedly. She does not remember that she broke both hips and had surgery.

Lately, she has been asking about her mother, who passed away in 2001. I tell her that her mother passed away at 86 years of age. Some days we will go over that topic several times in an hour.

It has been a journey since that first mini-stroke

LIVING IN THE MOMENT

in December 2006. When Aline was diagnosed with Alzheimer's in March 2009, I shared the news with the family. I had explained to them that one of the symptoms was memory loss and that the day would come when she would not recognize or remember us.

The next time our grandchildren were at the house, the youngest grandson said, "Nana, you still remember me, don't you?" Aline laughed, hugged him and replied, "I will always remember you."

However, I knew the day would indeed come when Aline would not remember us, but we would never forget her. She was a great wife, a great mother, and a great grandmother. She was the kindest, most loving, caring person I have ever known. She was loved by family and cherished by all her friends and colleagues.

Today, Aline is in the advanced stages, but she still recognizes family and some friends. She lives full time in a care facility, where our family continues their loving care for her.

Now, in Aline's name, I have a way to make a difference for others walking this path. The Aline Zerrenner Dementia Friendly Fund within the Community Foundation for the Fox Valley Region is propelling our dream of creating a dementia friendly community in the Fox Valley. My goal is to make it easy for people to obtain funding and not have to go through hoops for grants, and to have anyone be able to contribute to the fund.

On November 2, 2019, the first-ever Memory Café was held at the BEAMING Equine Therapy facility, funded by this charitable fund. Twenty-two people living with dementia and their caregivers participated in this interaction with therapy horses. Three more Memory Cafés were held at BEAMING.

COVID-19

In March 2020, Aline's care facility went into lockdown due to the spread of COVID-19. I was

LIVING IN THE MOMENT

unable to visit Aline until August when outside patio visits were allowed. I visited her three times, under strict COVID-19 guidelines, before the spike in the virus caused a second lockdown.

We communicated through notes, gifts, phone calls, and FaceTime. Aline was very confused by all this and it was difficult at times to communicate.

The staff has been fantastic during this pandemic with the care of all the residents. I am allowed to bring things to Aline and the staff delivers them to her. She received gifts from family for Mother's Day and her birthday. Staff also sends out weekly updates on the situation at the facility. The staff keeps me informed about any change in Aline and we have regularly scheduled care conference calls.

The men's support group that I facilitate resumed our monthly meetings while practicing safe social distancing and wearing masks. It is wonderful to have this group to share with each other and make the journey not so lonely.

These days, I pray that COVID-19 will soon pass and that I can continue "Living in the Moment" with Aline.

—*Walter Zerrenner ©2020*

LIVING IN THE MOMENT

"Continue to live in the moment."

A NOT SO LONELY JOURNEY

***"They are not giving you a hard time.
They are having a hard time."***

LOVE SURVIVES THE JOURNEY

On June 8, 2020, my wife and I "celebrated" our golden wedding anniversary. For the occasion, our kids contracted a sign company to put a large display on our front lawn for all the neighbors to see. Its message: "JUST MARRIED 50 YEARS AGO".

This year we also reached the sixteenth year of our journey with Alzheimer's Disease. It's hard to "celebrate" a golden wedding anniversary when one party has no memories of a marriage, of a life together, or even of a husband that she recognizes.

It feels a lot like losing your spouse, losing your culture, losing your life, your traditions and celebrations. It is unbelievable how important memory is to us humans.

A NOT SO LONELY JOURNEY

In the article "Long, Long Journey" published in the first book, *A Lonely Journey*, I chronicled the first 14 years of the journey with memory loss that my wife, Doris, and I have been living. In hindsight, those years seemed to be one challenge after another.

I've learned a lot. Perhaps the most revealing lesson has been that I, myself, am the greatest hurdle. Intellectually, I know that I can't blame Doris for her behavior or her anger, but emotionally I do. I tell myself she's not "trying" to give me a hard time; she's "having" a hard time. But my feelings are those of a husband whose wife is upset with him. My reactions to her anxiety have been the greatest hurdle I've had to overcome.

Since she has not recognized me as her husband the past couple of years, I've learned to see myself as her caregiver. I know it's a coping mechanism and I believe that's okay. So I tell myself that she is not angry with her husband, but with her caregiver.

And when she settles down, she really does love and care about her "caregiver."

I've learned that reasoning and pointing out reality such as "the roads are icy" is really arguing and it doesn't work. Neither do ultimatums such as "when you get dressed, we'll go."

Have you noticed when you give direction to accomplish a task, or to ask for cooperation, or to suggest a routine, that as you repeat yourself, your voice automatically gets more insistent and louder? And, of course, it doesn't work. I've found that it's better to whisper. A whisper draws her attention better than a directive or a demand. And it keeps the peace.

Communication is very difficult. Not only does Doris not understand what I say to her, I can't understand what she is trying to say, or asking about, and expecting an answer from me. She uses water for air, airplane for car, lake for snow, etc., etc. I try to pick out a word or phrase when I can catch one and I repeat it, or I say, "Yes" or "No" or "I don't know," in an attempt to keep her talking in order to have some semblance of a conversation.

Doris cannot answer my basic questions, "Are you hungry?" "Would you like…?" "Is it hot enough?" I have to taste her food to see if it's warm.

Caregiving is a heroic job. Besides learning to keep house, cook meals, do laundry, and give my wife my full attention when she is awake, I try to fit myself into her routine. Each day has different hours and routines.

Doris sleeps sixteen to eighteen hours a day at odd times. I have tried to eat meals with her, but she only eats once or twice a day. In the process, I've lost weight and cannot seem to regain it. I have come to realize that I need a schedule of three meals a day for myself, because, if my health goes down the river, we both drown.

I have also learned that I cannot walk this journey alone. However, asking for help is not an easy thing for a man to do. Over the past five years, my daughters, my sisters, and several home respite caregivers have allowed me the freedom to attend support groups. That has saved my life.

I have come to accept that I can't control so many things—what Doris will eat and when. How long she'll sleep or when she'll get up. If she'll put on her nightgown or sleep in her clothes. If she will get dressed when she rises, or insist we go for a car ride in her nightgown or bathrobe. Doris is frequently up in the middle of the night, hungry for breakfast at 2:00 a.m.

Since I've quit trying to control her routine, I'm more at peace. I am learning to "go with the flow." The old maxim is true, "You can lead a horse to water, but you can't make it drink."

It's hard to watch Doris mix her orange juice into her cereal, eat ice cream with her fingers, put lipstick in her hair (I've learned how to get that out), brush toothpaste on her forehead, put her nightgown or underwear in the toilet, and her soiled toilet paper in the waste basket. These things can't be corrected. She does not have the ability to learn.

Moodiness is part and parcel of this disease. I've sometimes described this life as living on "pins and needles." I am never sure when she'll get up or whether we can plan anything; if we will be able to make an event; if we will be on time as she does not have the ability to hurry; what kind of behavior she'll exhibit; or how she'll react to anything for no apparent reason.

Doris has a very short attention span. At this stage of her disease, within seconds or minutes of an anxious upset for unknown reasons, she can smile, put on a sweet expression, and even be very affectionate.

When she needs affection, she will give me a hug, and sometimes hang on and not want to let go. She will say, quite frequently now, "I love you very much." She has started to say, "I need you" and "I missed you." But within a short time she'll say, "Who are you?" My response, "John," seems to leave her confused.

Two years ago, I pulled out the love letters that we wrote to each other when we were courting. It proved to be a warm remembrance, but also a nostalgic grieving for the wife I had lost.

However, after that I began to treat her more like I did when we were courting—you know how you touch each other frequently. I consciously found opportunities to rub her back, to hold her hand, to give her hugs. She responded well to that.

Doris carries her "baby" doll with her most of the time. In the process of giving her baby affection, I give her affection. The loving compassion she has for her "baby" reminds me of the loving attention she gave to her five children when they were young.

I believe love is a choice. Love begins as a feeling, but soon you realize that love becomes a choice. Love is an action verb. You choose to prove your love by what you choose to do. When two people choose a mutual love, the feelings, the choosing, and the actions flow both ways. In such a mutual bond, the feelings, the choices, and the acts of love grow exponentially.

When one partner, in a growing and blossoming bond develops dementia, the reciprocal flow of energy and choice and action slowly fades. It is up to the caregiver partner to find ways to keep the flow, choices, and the actions going at least one way, even without the expectation of any reciprocation.

At that stage it may be hard to maintain the feelings of love, but the choices and the actions of love become even more important and more unselfish. For the person affected by the progressing memory loss, the choices and the actions of love become almost impossible. If you are lucky, there may be times when the love light in the eye glows for a moment and the feelings can still be expressed.

I have learned to cherish those moments and those feelings, because they will have to compensate for the times when the brain is unable to make loving choices or to perform loving actions.

Because of my poor hearing, I tend to watch people's lips in order to lip read. But recently I've concentrated on looking into Doris' eyes. She responds to that. She looks me straight in the eye, gets a twinkle in her eyes and smiles. It is like seeing into her soul.

Doris is still my wife. I am so grateful that she is still with me, day by day, no matter her many changes in behavior and loss of ability to communicate or to care for herself. She is the same woman I married 50 years ago.

We will never get back to a life of blissful "peace and harmony," but I can give her "moments of joy" such as car rides which are soothing and therapeutic for her. We go for rides every day, usually for several hours.

After 16 years of dementia caregiving, I hope that I am starting to get the knack of this, but I still make mistakes every day. I catch myself trying to use reality—my reality. But at least I catch myself. I'm learning to set aside my emotions and my natural instinct of reacting. I'm learning to slow down, to give her time to putter, to lay aside my drive for efficiency and control of every situation. I'm trying to let her dictate the flow of our day.

We have a bedtime ritual each night. No matter how upset she may have been that day or how resistive she may have been to going to bed, once I help her into bed, her face brightens and she smiles at me. I give her a foot massage. I hug her. I say, "Good night, sleep tight, don't let the bed bugs bite" and then I kiss both her and the "baby" on the cheek. I then say, "I love you" and kiss her on the lips. She returns the kiss and says, "I love you very much." I rub her back, her shoulder, her arm, and tuck her in for the night. She closes her eyes and falls peacefully asleep almost instantly. It's a ritual that does both our hearts good. That's our celebration of a golden anniversary every day.

—John Weyers ©2020

"It provides interaction between us."

MY DAY AS A CAREGIVER

The world changed on 9/11. In trying to keep a schedule for Tom's bodily functions, I tell him it's time to get up at 8:30 a.m. He has the choice of a shower today or tomorrow. He picks tomorrow.

As we walk down the hallway to the dining room table, I wonder to myself, when did he get so stooped over? He was taller than I, but we are now the same height.

Tom always does his diabetes check before he eats or takes his pills. This is always a test of my patience, but I allow him to do the diabetes routine himself.

Even though his zippered container is at his place, he starts to sit in another chair. He opens his smaller zippered pouch and stops. "Test strips," I remind him. He takes out more than he needs and shuts the container. He inserts the test strip in the tester correctly today. I then point to the poker with the needle that is used to draw blood. He pokes a finger near the nail, and while squeezing it to draw blood, he rubs the blood off. When a drop of blood is formed on another finger after another poke, he does not allow the blood to flow to the end of the test strip. The error message appears. Still another poke, and another squeeze, and the blood on a new test strip prompts the success message. Tom then records the number where I indicate it should go.

I ask him, "If yesterday was 9-10, then what is today?" He knows and writes 9-11, but he forgets the stem on the 9 so it looks like a zero.

His injection pen is on the table. I ask, "How much do you give yourself?" He answers, "Forty-four" and the dial is turned to that number.

I take the needle out of his pouch and Tom attaches it onto the pen. He removes the needle cover. He needs a reminder to pull down his pajamas so he sees his abdomen and doesn't inject through the cloth. With hesitation, he pushes the pen and releases the Lantus. Now the needle needs to come off. After several attempts, I do it for him.

Things need to be put away. Extra test strips are picked up, but the container is closed so the test strips fall. The container is opened. Strips are picked up one by one and aligned. Finally, the test strips are placed in the open container and with my direction, the rest of the items are put away. Yes, it would be easier to do it myself, but it is one of the few things he can still do with direction. It also provides interaction between us.

Tom no longer initiates conversation. At this point with directions, his other self sufficient activities of daily living are dressing and undressing, showering, tying his shoes, shaving with an electric razor, brushing his teeth, getting in and out of a chair, eating, sometimes fastening and unfastening his seat belt. Patience.

Many times, toileting is the task family caregivers can't handle. We normally spend the summer at our cottage where we do not have a washing machine. The cottage was built in the 1940s and there is no place to put one. Nursing homes use two hour intervals for toileting. During the month of August, I was toileting Tom day and night. Tom wears pull-ups, but sometimes the bed gets wet. Bowel accidents happen too, but with a shower the care is now routine.

Sleep is Tom's activity of choice. Memory Cafés, choir, and SPARK programs used to get both of us out of the house. We use Zoom meetings now due to COVID-19. For a time, we had to drive to our public library parking lot to use their Internet on our smart phone. Now we have Internet service at our home and use the computer for the Zoom meetings. Tom smiles when he sees familiar faces and responds to questions if I repeat the question.

MY DAY AS A CAREGIVER

Not many of Tom's friends are left as he is 92 years old. One childhood friend calls him about once a month and reminisces about their childhood neighborhood. Several friends have visited while sitting on chairs in our driveway with masks and social distancing.

It is a remarriage for both of us. Several of his five children and in-laws are wonderful about contacting him and visiting. My family is closer in miles so their contact with both of us is easier. Again, it's masks and distancing and no more than two other adults inside.

Tom stays awake and appears to listen. He smiles appropriately and will respond to questions. The questions are usually choice questions such as, "Would you like a ham or turkey sandwich?"

So another day in another week, another month, another year. Sometimes "same old, same old" can be a comfort. There are no surprises, no health difficulties. We are grateful for what we continue to have.

Recently, Tom fell after he lost his balance getting up from a chair. He fell on the living room carpet and hit the coffee table breaking four ribs and bruising his left lung. He was hospitalized as the lung needed draining.

Tom had a definite personality change several days before that. He had told me to shut up. This was not Tom who has maintained an old world courtesy—"please" and "thank you" always. Tom even cleared his throat and spit in an inappropriate place.

In the hospital, Tom was walking for about 150 feet with a walker in the hallway while wearing a mask. Meals were eaten in a chair, and infrequently he sat on the toilet. His activity of choice was sleeping, which seemed to be a necessity, not just a choice. He was impossible to wake up at times so therapy would often be canceled.

Covid has made a difference in his recovery as

I perceive it. Except for two days, I was allowed to be with him during his hospital stay. Staff usually tried to accommodate my wishes for both physical and occupational therapy. A gait belt was used to help him get out of bed, to move to the chair, and for safety while walking. A catheter was inserted to get a urine sample as he was incontinent, and tests showed that he did have a urinary tract infection.

Broken ribs are painful, but the pain was handled well using a Q catheter which released pain medication to the site instead of using a systemic pain killer. The lung drainage tube was removed before he left the hospital as well as the Q catheter.

Finding a rehab place for him was not easy as my places of choice would not take him due to the pandemic. We found an excellent rated nursing rehab facility which provided transportation to their facility. Tom rode in the van in a wheelchair and I followed in our car. Due to the pandemic, Wisconsin nursing homes currently have a 14 day quarantine for new admissions. That meant Tom had to stay in his room for his first 14 days there.

Fortunately, after a few glitches, the staff arranged some FaceTime sessions for us. I didn't realize how hard it is to be interactive with a person for 15 minutes who responds only with a "yes" or "no." Sometimes sleep took over and I would just watch Tom drop his head and nod off.

A care conference was held after the quarantine was lifted and I was asked to write down what Tom would need to be able to do before he could come home.

Two doctor visits were scheduled outside the facility, but each would have resulted in another 14 day quarantine upon his return. I took the responsibility for canceling them. At this point, he may need further drainage of the left lung, but that remains to be seen.

Now we are able to "window time" for 15 minutes daily which gives me a chance to see all of him, not just his face. I read letters to Tom and show him cards that he has received. A delightful card from a granddaughter talked about things she remembered about him such as eating black bananas, wearing plaid Christmas pants, and giving fun money for birthdays.

I have noticed Tom is not able to reach the floor with his feet due to the seat cushion in his wheelchair. He needs the cushion because of the breakdown of the skin on his buttocks. He cannot maneuver the chair with his feet and he does not know how to use his hands to propel it.

His left leg is swollen. Is that from falls that he has had? He was found sitting on the foot pedals of his wheelchair and sitting on the floor in front of his lounge chair. He had two clots in his leg years ago. Is this the precursor to another one? He says there is no pain in his leg or ribs. Is that true? From seeing his reaction in the hospital, I do think he registers pain, but would he remember that something bothered him? From having hands, eyes and ears on Tom 24/7, I am frustrated by the lack of contact. My consolation is that the staff seem caring and considerate.

Will Tom be able to come home? I don't know. I do know there is an overwhelming silence when a person is missing. I am experiencing frustration, acceptance, and sadness.

—*Jean Orbison* ©2020

MY DAY AS A CAREGIVER

"Grateful for what we continue to have."

A NOT SO LONELY JOURNEY

"I am human."

NOT DOING ENOUGH

My husband, David, was diagnosed with dementia in 2012. It still feels like yesterday that we were sitting in the psychologist's office awaiting the results of the testing. I remember thinking, "Just say it! Just tell us the results!" We had been dealing with the unknown way too long and even waited months for the appointment.

Finally, she told us he definitely had some form of dementia, but they would need more time and testing to narrow it down. She told us that at this point, the tests were not indicative of Alzheimer's disease. I was told to bring David back in a year so they could do a comparison test which may help to narrow his diagnosis down further. I was somewhat relieved to have the dementia diagnosis as other doctors had been looking at a mental health diagnosis. An MRI was also ordered to create a baseline as well as to help confirm the diagnosis.

At the time, David was in his early fifties. I had heard of early onset dementia, sometimes referred to as young onset dementia, which is a term used when a person is younger than 65 years old. At a dementia conference, I met a woman, who was 32, and cared for her husband who was diagnosed with early onset dementia. They had two small children. My heart went out to her and it made me count my blessings.

Of course, I researched and read everything I could get my hands on trying to figure out exactly what dementia we were dealing with. Doctors have told me it is important to know what we were dealing with due to possible side effects and interaction with David's other medications. With all my research, I was feeling like a medical student as well as an expert on dementia—if there is such a thing.

Besides having to change directions, especially with our retirement dreams, I found it most aggravating that family, friends, and even strangers seemed to want to "help." Their definition of help, however, was to tell me what I should or should not be doing. What I was hearing was that I was doing it all wrong!

Probably the most frustrating situations are when people ask me if I really think the test results are accurate and that I should get (yet) another opinion. Didn't they have any idea how relieved I was to have somewhat of a "label" for what David was experiencing? Some would even comment they didn't see anything wrong or different with David. I often took these comments to mean something must be wrong with me! Deep down, I know they were trying to truly help, but it only added to my anxiety. Recalling these situations still makes me fume.

Don't they know that I already doubt myself a hundred times a day wondering if I am doing enough? What else can I possibly do? I pray for a cure. I pray for him to get better. Am I praying for the wrong things? I do know my own wellness is suffering and that I need to work more on my self-doubt.

As difficult as it is, I am learning to ignore those who do not have medical degrees or experience in caring for a person with a dementia diagnosis. I simply change the subject. Most get my message, but there are always a few who are oblivious and I have to be more direct. I try my best not to be rude, but sometimes it is difficult to hold back.

I want everyone to know that I have been, and continue to do everything possible to get David the best possible care. Unless you have actually walked in the shoes of a family caregiver, don't critique my care or my love for David. You cannot possibly know the challenges I, or other family caregivers, deal with on a daily basis.

If you really want to help me, give me words of encouragement. Give me a hug. Tell me I am doing a great job of caring for David. If you cannot be sincere, then please say nothing. I do not want your pity. I can already see your pity reflected in your eyes.

David is no longer capable of expressing any appreciation or love for me. Any recognition from you for a sincere "job well done" is extremely appreciated. An in-law, who has since passed, would approach me at family gatherings and she would give me a hug and thank me for taking such good care of David. I miss her.

I am human. Yes, I often wear a smile and a brave face when you see me, but know that I have my moments too. Your positive support means so much to me and to David as well.

—*Anna* ©2020

"You will land on your feet."

NOW WHAT?

The doctor just told you the test results indicate cognitive impairment. Further testing will be needed, but Alzheimer's is suspected. Now what?

I admit, I was stunned even though the results were what I expected for my husband. So many decisions to make in so many areas in such a short amount of time. I knew he would most definitely have to quit his job as he has been struggling at work. I realized I would also have to resign my job as well to care for him. How would we manage? Could we afford to keep the house? Neither of us were retirement age. Why couldn't it have just been a benign tumor the doctors could remove and everything would be fine?

It felt my researching and reading everything

I could find on dementia became my life. Are there new medications that may slow or reverse the disease? What type of diet could help? What activities could help? I was frustrated with the lack of answers.

I decided to get my husband involved in some memory-based group activities. He wasn't interested and after several attempts refused to attend anymore. I, however, found the interaction with other family caregivers was just what I needed.

I did more research and found a few caregiver support groups in my area. New friends that really understand what it is like to be a family caregiver with no judgment. This is what I needed! What I have learned and continue to learn from these fellow caregivers is truly priceless. I believe the support and sharing of knowledge that I receive from other caregivers makes me a better caregiver for my husband.

NOW WHAT

In looking back, I have to say everything worked out considering the circumstances. Yes, I had plenty of sleepless nights with worry, but somehow, we landed on our feet. I admit it took time, but I assure you that you will eventually land on your feet as well.

—Suzanna ©2020

A NOT SO LONELY JOURNEY

"I no longer feel alone."

OUR JOURNEY

I think back to our life before brain disease became our focus. We had a good life. We had a good marriage. I was working five to seven days a week. The work was fun and exciting. I was making more money than at any time in my life.

Martha was my partner. She took care of my office and our home. She was organized and in control of everything we needed to be successful. In another 8 to 10 years, we expected to retire.

We planned to buy a two-seat sports car and travel the country a few months each year. We hoped to have fun and enjoy having more control over our life. We had plans and dreams. Life was good.

Then Martha started having problems. She

would trip and fall. She was sometimes agitated and angry. We thought the medicine she was taking for bipolar was causing side effects. We started looking for answers. We went to a variety of doctors: general practitioners, psychiatrists, and neurologists. We were frustrated. It took almost three years to finally begin to understand what was happening to her.

At the same time, Martha was really struggling physically and emotionally. Two examples of these struggles changed everything. First, she hit her head on the wall inside the front door closet when she tripped over the threshold coming into the house. Second, Martha broke her shoulder when she fell off the bed. We knew we had to find answers to this illness. The frustration grew as we kept seeing more doctors.

We finally received a dual diagnosis of vascular dementia and normal pressure hydrocephalus. What? I had never heard of these diseases. I had no idea how much our lives were going to change beyond what we had already experienced.

Martha and I worked to adapt to the changes in her physical ability and cognitive challenges. The cognitive issues were manageable. She could not help me at work much anymore, so we adjusted our way of doing things. I thought we could stay with the plan to continue working until we were 70.

However, Martha's health continued to decline. We were now dealing with strokes. She would get lost when she drove, or when she walked alone, and she had problems handling finances. She would sometimes even take the wrong medications.

After three trips to the emergency room, doctors told me not to bring her in for strokes as there was nothing they could do for her except make her comfortable and wait a few hours. Instead, they educated me on how to care for her at home.

Martha's cognitive abilities continued to decline. At this point, she could no longer drive, leave home alone, handle money, or medications. We tried neurosurgery and had a shunt implanted with the hope of reversing the physical symptoms of the normal pressure of hydrocephalus. It didn't work.

At the same time, we were getting plenty of advice from lots of people on what else we should be doing. Most of the advice was not helpful. Even doctors did not know how to help. We were mostly on our own in this battle and found that even adapting and changing did not really help much. We were fighting a battle we could not win.

This was new to me. In the past, I had been able to solve our problems. I worked hard at my job. I worked hard to have a good family, a happy family.

Martha and I had always figured out what to do when difficulties happened. I worked hard and fixed most problems. Now, I didn't know how to fix Martha's health. I felt lost. I felt incompetent. I am a man, husband and father. I am supposed to be able to fix this. I couldn't.

Realizing that I could not fix what was wrong with Martha was difficult. I had to figure out what I could do because I wanted to take care of her and protect her.

I realized I needed to quit my job. I was determined to find a way to help Martha. We read books. We went to see specialists. We applied through our local Aging and Disability Resource Center (ADRC) for help. We kept asking questions. Sometimes we weren't sure we were asking the right questions. Mostly, we didn't know what was available or even who to ask for help.

Then we found the Fox Valley Memory Project. We went to a few Memory Cafés where we met people who knew what we were going through. They were actually able to help us understand what was happening to us. We received good advice based on facts and experience. These people cared about us. They were strangers who were willing and able to help us on this new journey.

We had to accept a whole new way of life that was so different from anything we had dreamed of living. We could never have planned for this journey, but now we had help that could truly make a difference for us. They helped me see that I was still thinking I had to fix Martha. I realized I had to keep asking for help and learn what I could do for Martha that would truly help.

During this time, Martha and I were together all day every day. I had started to think I was not doing enough because her health was getting worse, not better. I worried every day about her falling. I spent a lot of my time trying to figure out what else I could do to help her. I felt helpless. I felt like I was failing. I knew I had to find help. I felt like the problems I faced were overwhelming. I felt lost in this new world of dementia. I also felt that God was not helping us. Talk about feeling alone! I was pushing God away too.

Then I was introduced to a man at a Memory Café. He and his wife had been on their journey through the world of dementia for about 12 years. He facilitated a support group for husbands who are caregivers for their wives. It was obvious now that something had to change.

I started attending the support group and began learning the truth about dementia. I learned the truth about what I could and could not do. I started to feel better. Maybe God was helping after all. I had found other men who knew what I was feeling.

The details of our journeys were different for each of us, but now I was not alone on the path. These were men I could trust. They cared about me. They gave me their time and emotional support to help me understand how to care for my wife and for myself along the way.

Now, I no longer felt so alone. I knew our

children and friends cared about us. I knew they were doing their best for us, but in the daily struggle of life, we were alone. They could not possibly know what it was like for me as I tried to help Martha. They could not understand how I felt all alone in this struggle.

The support group men could relate to and understand my struggles. They helped me know what the future was going to be like. I no longer felt alone on this difficult journey. I knew, that as men and husbands, they had also felt helpless and alone just like me. I no longer felt like a failure. God helped me find this group of men.

I was now able to ask the right questions of people who could help us. I realized it is okay to not know what to do. I had to let go of my need to fix everything. I found a way to have caregivers come to the house daily to help Martha. I learned what I can and cannot change.

I was excited by what I was learning. I wanted

to better understand what I could do, so I asked the facilitator if we could meet for coffee as I wanted more information. We met between the monthly support group meetings and have become close friends.

He and the rest of the guys helped me to stop feeling sorry for myself. I had not realized how guilty I was feeling for not being able to fix Martha. Guilt had made me feel very sorry for myself.

Today, I still go to the support group. The facilitator has become my best friend. We have lunch together and play golf. We can laugh and have fun. That group of men, and especially the facilitator, have changed my life. My journey is not so lonely now. I thank God always for helping me find caring men who know what I'm feeling and thinking. I smile more now.

This journey inside the world of dementia has helped me look at my life differently. No more guilt and self-pity, at least most of the time. I am still

A NOT SO LONELY JOURNEY

very sad at times and so is Martha, but that's okay. We can also find things to smile and laugh about in this life.

—George Butz ©2020

"Find things to laugh about."

A NOT SO LONELY JOURNEY

"Together we have it all."

OUR LIFE PUZZLE

If you would have asked me 15 years ago what I pictured my life to be like, a young and in love 18-year-old would have said, "The future looks bright!" If you ask me the same question today, at age 34 and married for almost 14 years, my answer would sound much different.

My life feels like a jigsaw puzzle, but with a few missing pieces. I live day to day, and sometimes minute to minute, carefully trying to piece together the intricate pieces of this puzzle I call life.

Little did I know when I married Bryan, I was not only claiming the title of "wife," but also "advocate, supporter, champion, breadwinner, caregiver, detective, and critic" to name just a few. These additional roles were not exactly what I envisioned as we stood at the altar and vowed to love each other "for better or for worse."

Given I was pursuing a college degree in social work, at that time, I felt the Lord was leading me toward a life of service both in my career and in my family life. I dove into my newfound role with confidence that I would show my love by assuring Bryan felt happy, loved, and supported. I put my whole heart and soul into this man that I love so very much.

Despite the challenges that were put in front of us, we were on top of the world feeling like we could take on anything that came our way. Little did I know this was only the beginning of a long journey.

Our journey started shortly after graduating from high school in the summer of 2005. Bryan and I had been high school friends, but "friend" isn't exactly how I was feeling. So, I regularly stopped into the local A&W when I saw his familiar truck in the parking lot to eat their famous cheese fries.

Several weeks after graduation, we both found ourselves single and began spending more and more time together. I quickly fell in love and wanted to spend every waking moment with him.

As we headed into fall, I went off to college while Bryan was finalizing his plans to enlist in the United States Marine Corps, just as his grandfather and father had done. We knew it would be a challenge maintaining a long-distance relationship, that goes hand and hand with military family life, but we were committed to stick together and see where our relationship would take us.

Bryan left for basic training at the Marine Corps Recruit Depot (MCRD) in San Diego, California on January 11, 2006. This date will always stick out in my mind, due to the effort it appeared that I took to see him just one more time before he left.

It was a snowy morning and I was running late on my morning commute to school. I found myself sliding off the road and into a ditch. I tearfully called Bryan to tell him what happened. He and his dad came to my rescue a short time later. I will never live it down that I had purposely landed in the ditch just so that I could see Bryan one more time before he left for 12 weeks.

Over the next few weeks, Bryan's parents allowed me to stay in his room to find comfort in his absence. I happened to be at their house, between my school and work commitments the last week of January, when the phone rang. It was Bryan.

My initial reaction was one of fear due to having been told by his recruiter that contact with family comes in stages while in basic training. We were still in the letter writing phase. Bryan's Mom and I both picked up the phone and listened as Bryan, between sobs, informed us that he had been diagnosed with a brain tumor.

He further explained that during the past few weeks, his drill instructors earmarked him under the assumption that he was not paying attention during drills. His vision was checked and appeared to be within normal limits, except for some concerns about his peripheral vision. This resulted in further evaluation at a naval medical center to rule out any other contributing conditions that may be causing vision changes.

The rest of the conversation is a blur to me. Questions ran through my mind: "What will happen next? Will they send him home? How are they going to treat this?" In a matter of hours, Bryan's family and I had booked our plane tickets. By the next week we were on a plane to San Diego to find out what the next steps were.

After many evaluation/diagnostic exams, we learned that Bryan was diagnosed with a rare brain tumor, optic nerve glioma, which involves the optic nerve and optic chiasm. The initial plan was set for Bryan to have surgery to remove what was feasible of his tumor. Doctors also planned to do a complete biopsy during surgery to determine their next steps. Despite the urgency of the surgery, it was delayed due to Bryan having a sinus infection. The surgery was rescheduled for mid-March 2006.

After several weeks in California and now knowing the anticipated plan for surgery, I tearfully returned home to tend to my school and work obligations. I longed to be comforting Bryan, but the reality of the situation was that I needed to continue moving forward with my life and educational goals despite this devastating news.

The days were long, and I filled my time with work and school to avoid the painful thoughts and questions that came to mind when I had idle time. Community members and local church congregations added Bryan to their prayer lists.

Despite the overwhelming support, I continued to worry amidst unanswered questions as we prepared for the surgery. Through the hard times, reminders of God's presence surrounded us as others stepped in when we needed it most.

Bryan's gunnery sergeant and his wife and their children became our second family and still are today. They truly were our angels along this journey. We were welcomed into their home with open arms. They provided home cooked meals and transportation around San Diego. Most of all, they helped us grow deeper in our faith during a time when we needed this hope the most. We are truly blessed that God sent us these angels in our time of need!

I returned to California the week prior to Bryan's surgery. Despite being a recruit, which are typically not allowed off base, Bryan was granted privileges off base to spend time with his family. We visited the San Diego Zoo, Balboa Park, the beach, and simply enjoyed time together.

The day of the surgery came. We prayed for the best outcome as we watched them wheel Bryan off to surgery. All we could think about were the possible outcomes of the surgery such as brain damage, vision loss, paralysis, personality or behavioral changes, and even death. The possibilities were unbearable. The estimated length of the surgery was unknown, but we were informed Bryan could be in surgery for over 24 hours depending on what was found during the surgery.

We waited hour after hour and received surgery updates every couple of hours. After almost eight hours of surgery, one of the doctors came out to the waiting room and took Bryan's parents and I back to a room to explain what they had found.

The type of brain tumor they had discovered was not what they had initially thought. The brain tumor was growing out of his optic nerve and crossing into his other optic nerve. Since they could not differentiate the tumor from his optic nerve, the only option would be to halt the surgery and come back together as a team, including Bryan, to determine a treatment plan. If they continued to remove the tumor, they would be removing his optic nerves causing total and permanent vision loss.

Bryan's neurosurgeon was considered to be one of the leading specialists in the field. The neurosurgeon explained that his medical team would meet with Bryan and us in the coming days to gain consent from Bryan. This would allow them to move forward with the removal that would leave him blind and faced with the reality that he and his family would need to start learning Braille.

As we learned Bryan's fate, we knew our lives would be changing forever. Naive to the ways of the world and the direct impact that this would have on Bryan, I can look back now and realize that my selfish disappointments and feelings in those moments paled in comparison to the 180 degree direction change for Bryan. His life was turning upside down. At that moment, he didn't even know it yet.

Prior to the next team meeting, Bryan's neurosurgeon further researched this specific tumor. We met again within a few days to follow up on his findings. He had consulted with a Mayo Clinic neurosurgeon and scanned medical journals to find effective treatment options. He discovered Bryan's brain tumor was unique in that this tumor is primarily found in babies and children under 10 years of age. Bryan was one of only a small number of adults found to have this type of tumor. Despite the tumor being slow growing and Bryan having had it since birth, treatment was still necessary to stop the continued growth.

Research pointed to radiation as the best course of treatment given the limited information they had to base their decisions. The treatment plan was made. Appointments were scheduled with doctors and social workers to plan a successful surgery and recovery. Thankfully, my spring break happened to fall within this time period which allowed me to extend my stay in California to continue helping Bryan through his recovery.

After Bryan was transferred out of ICU, he went to the Neurosurgery Unit where he started inpatient rehabilitation for speech, physical, and occupational therapy. It was only a matter of days before it became clear that Bryan was not recovering at the rate of most individuals who have undergone brain surgery.

I can recall one specific incident when Bryan complained of pain after being woken up by a nurse. She advised him that he had just received his pain medication and was not due for more. She proceeded to assist him up and tell him that he was going to go for a walk. Bryan did as he was told, but it was obvious that he could not walk without a two person assist. At that point. the nurse pointed out another male patient who had only just come out of brain surgery one day prior. He was already out of bed showing his efforts towards recovery.

My heart felt sad for Bryan and angry at the nurse for not showing empathy to a young man, only 19 years old, who was recently informed of his life-threatening illness. Bryan was also dealing with an ever-evolving treatment plan in a state halfway across the country from his home and away from the support of friends and family.

It was from this point that I made a commitment to myself to make sure that I did everything within my power, and for as long as I was able, to ensure Bryan was well cared for, his voice was heard, his concerns taken seriously, and that he understood how much he was valued.

After several more days and limited progress in his daily therapies, Bryan was discharged from the rehab floor. He returned to his medical hold platoon housing located on the hospital campus ground to continue his recovery.

His family and I had been staying at the Fisher House, similar to the Ronald McDonald House, which proved to be a godsend. They provided our housing and food needs at no cost to us due to the generous donation of others.

It was less than 12 hours when the call came at 5 a.m. that Bryan was currently in the ER, had been intubated, and was undergoing further evaluation after he was found having a seizure on the bathroom floor. Panic ensued when the reality set in that having undergone brain surgery recently, there were many factors to rule out the cause of the seizures, none of which I wanted to think about. This period of time remains a blur.

Bryan was stabilized and the seizure activity controlled. Following many tests, it was found that Bryan had bacterial meningitis. The doctors struggled to understand how this could have occurred, but informed us that the only likely cause is that he acquired the bacterial infection during his recent brain surgery. This diagnosis further explained his symptoms, complaints, and uncharacteristically long recovery time since his initial surgery.

The profound gravity of a meningitis diagnosis has only just started to sink in as I write this. Bryan was very sick for quite some time. He had numerous days in a row with only brief periods of being awake, and incoherent speech when he attempted to communicate.

Thinking back, I was so focused on the brain tumor with trying to understand the treatment options, that any secondary diagnoses or issues paled in comparison to what I understood to be the primary issue that needed to be dealt with. My sole focus was to get through the medical treatment necessary to get rid of this tumor, so that we could get back home and start our life together and put all of this behind us.

Within a short time, Bryan was back in the operating room undergoing his second brain surgery in a matter of weeks. This time the team included an infectious disease specialist, to determine the extent of the bacterial meningitis infection, assess his brain function, determine if any damage had occurred, and as the doctors explained, "disinfect Bryan's brain and the bone pieces that were cut during his first surgery" in an attempt to minimize the spread of the infection.

Bryan came out of surgery with promising news that the meningitis had not infected his brain or surrounding tissue ruling out the possibility of him contracting this during his surgery. It remains a mystery how the infection entered his body.

After surgery, Bryan was started on strong antibiotics that required placement of a PICC line to be able to easily administer the medication multiple times per day over the course of eight weeks to treat the infection. While receiving his course of antibiotics, Bryan continued to see specialists in the fields of radiology, endocrinology, ophthalmology, and neuropsychology. His radiation treatment was delayed by eight weeks so that Bryan could finish a full antibiotics course for treatment of meningitis.

Throughout this time, I was keeping up-to-date on Bryan's latest developments through daily phone calls with his parents. He would also occasionally call me, but since he was still considered "property of the government," Bryan could only make calls when he was granted privileges.

Bryan began to learn his fate during meeting after meeting with specialists advising of the impending risks, likely side effects of radiation, his prognosis, and future follow up needed. At the time, Bryan was living in a world of medical terminology while his parents stepped in to assist in making decisions that would inevitably impact his future forever.

Our relationship was thriving despite the chaos. We were living on young teenage love, occasional phone calls, and giddy excitement in anticipation of seeing each other again. We could forget about the current situation and just enjoy spending time with each other. We looked to the future, excitedly planned our future children's names, and thrived on the hope that our life would be seamless once we were able to get past this one hurdle.

Due to the location of the tumor and targeted radiation site, it was impossible to avoid radiating the hypothalamus which is the message control sender for sending hormones to the pituitary glands. The effects would cause chronic lifelong challenges that would require frequent follow up appointments to monitor his hormones and provide synthetic hormones for his body to function. The doctors advised us that in post treatment, the chances of conceiving naturally would be slim due to low testosterone levels that would further be impacted by radiation.

Bryan was just 19 years old, but the radiologist asked us if we had discussed family planning or the timing of children. The best chances for naturally conceiving a child would be in the eight weeks prior to the start of his radiation treatment. In the blink of an eye, we went from the biggest decision we had to make was the restaurant choice for dinner to now deciding if we wanted children. We seemed to be doing well with all that was coming at us as we continued to live in our own fairy tale, and the false reality that we could accomplish anything if we still had each other. Additional steps were taken to assure that sperm was banked so that with further medical intervention, the possibility of having children still existed if we so chose.

Thinking back to the late night conversations with my parents, before Bryan and I were married, I now understand why my parents wanted to make sure that I truly understood the level of commitment I was undertaking. They knew and understood that marriage was hard work and that Bryan and I would have an extra layer of difficulty with his diagnosis of a brain tumor resulting in traumatic brain injury (TBI) from his course of treatment and lasting side effects.

As a young adult just barely out of high school, my small worldview could not even comprehend that we would be anything but happy. His diagnosis was only a speed bump that would help us to grow stronger having gone through this together.

At the end of May, close to the end of Bryan's six-week course of radiation treatment, I was able to visit him once again. It was on this trip, May 22, 2006, that Bryan made it official by asking the long-awaited question, "Will you marry me?" I knew we were destined to live out our "forever after" based on the time and effort Bryan had spent planning every girl's dream proposal, all while undergoing the biggest challenge of his life.

The evening was complete with a limousine tour of downtown San Diego with stops at monumental landmarks, the most amazing Italian dinner, and a sunset walk on Coronado Island Beach—which is where I was certain would be the moment he was going to pop the question, but much to my surprise and disappointment, he didn't. Our tour ended that night with a walk through the Medical Center Healing Garden which led to a waterfall covered in mini floating tea light candles—about 100 of them. Bryan got down on one knee. It was the most romantic, thoughtful proposal and I couldn't think of any other person I wanted to spend the rest of my life with.

On June 14, 2006, Bryan was finally able to return home to Wisconsin. The anticipation of him finally coming home to stay was filled with overwhelming joy and excitement. Underneath this happiness remained a sense of fear of the unknowns the future would bring. Our life as an engaged couple began, but the excitement was short lived as we delved into the overwhelming process of navigating the Veterans healthcare system and the seemingly endless medical appointments and evaluations to establish medical care in Wisconsin. Not to mention the complex task of determining program eligibility for military programs, short term disability, insurance benefits, etc.

I cannot recall the exact time it dawned on me that the life I had imagined of establishing my career, beginning our family, placing my career on hold in order to be home with our babies, and returning to work once our children were school age, would remain an intangible dream. If I were to be in this relationship for the long term, I would have to decide to let go of the expectations that I had for my family and transition to primary breadwinner.

Without the assistance of knowledgeable professionals, most notably our local Veterans Service Officer, we would not be where we are today. He was instrumental in using his resources to get Bryan a service connected disability compensation. He meticulously fought for Bryan to receive a permanent and total service-connected disability rating. His advocacy was truly amazing. I especially value his exceptional commitment now that I have been in the social work field for over 10 years and seeing the bureaucratic red tape that presents barriers to situations such as ours.

Since we began our life together in 2006, we have been through a multitude of life obstacles both in our relationship and with medical events, including multiple seizure episodes which are now controlled through medication. However, not before Bryan was let go from his job due to being considered a liability risk after having a seizure on the job.

Over the years, all the medical challenges Bryan endured have taken a toll on his overall wellbeing. I have observed Bryan struggle with severe depression and anxiety with the inability to control what is happening to him. His short-term memory impairments are evident, and strategies to manage this include notebooks scattered all over our home and vehicles, only for Bryan to forget where he left them lay. Feelings of inadequacy flood his everyday thoughts despite my offering encouragement and hope. As much as Bryan loves his children, I can see that his being a stay at home dad was not the future he envisioned. He would much rather be working to provide for our family.

The most challenging part of our life has been experiencing the many trials and challenges which have forced us to adjust or let go of the expectations that we may have had for our family. Personally, I struggle every day with feelings of inadequacy due to my fear of being unable to keep our family's life in order, which I fail to do time and time again. Initially I put on a good front, but it didn't take long for the control I thought I had, to turn into a primary stressor in our marriage.

Year after year, I have taken on more and more household responsibilities to lessen the stress and responsibility for Bryan. I could never have imagined that my idea of helping could be viewed as anything other than that.

During one of my darkest seasons, I had very little hope. I couldn't see any light at the end of the road no matter what path I traveled. It was then that a good friend reached out to me and shared a Focus on the Family Broadcast from April 2017, in which the featured author, Laura Story, discussed in her book, "When God Doesn't Fix It." She shared her personal story of marriage and family life amidst her husband's chronic illness.

After learning of her family's journey and how uncannily similar her story is to Bryan's and mine, it brought hope that I desperately needed. I felt that I was no longer alone in my struggles. A glimpse into Laura's raw, honest emotions from the good, the bad, to the ugly, allowed me to let go of most of the guilt and resentment I had been holding onto. With time, I'm learning to forgive myself for the things I have thought, the hurtful things I have said, and the actions that have been selfish or childish.

Living with my husband's memory loss, variable moods, hormone changes, cognitive deficits, speech difficulty, and mental health challenges, has brought about unique challenges in how we live our day to day lives.

My mother would confirm that I have always lacked patience since I was a little girl. I am a type A personality that is motivated with a "get 'er done" type of attitude. I keep busy and typically don't know what to do with myself when I have down time. As you can imagine, this is contrary to living with an individual with disabilities.

Life is just a bit harder, with unanticipated surprises, and little ability to plan far into the future or even sometimes the next day. I like to think that God has a sense of humor when he decided that Bryan was to be my life partner, knowing that I had a lot to learn to be able to slow down and enjoy life's journey. I continue to receive daily reminders of the importance of developing patience when I'm presented with unanticipated schedule changes or interruptions during our daily routines.

One might take an outside look at our family and see a typical family life. However, without knowing Bryan and our story, one would not be able to identify the "silent disability" that has proven to be a primary staple in our life. Bryan is very social and likeable, which is a strength of his. But to his disadvantage, others do not understand the challenges he endures. Since he appears so "normal" during brief conversational exchanges, others do not see the challenges behind his personable smile and witty sense of humor.

Previously, I hated meeting new people because it gave me anxiety to have to explain Bryan's story and the unique roles we each serve in our family. A simple question of, "What does your husband do for a living?" causes my stomach to turn as I know, all too well, the awkwardness that will soon follow.

There are also the uncomfortable moments of silence that occur when Bryan is unable to recall the words that he is trying to say. The long pauses when Bryan is struggling to get the words from his brain to his mouth. I often want to just finish his sentences to avoid this inevitable awkwardness. This limitation is only compounded by my past insensitivity of telling Bryan that he was "socially awkward."

My immaturity and lack of impulse control during times of frustration and stress has created many regrets and added guilt for myself. It is only within the past year that Bryan has shared how frustrating it is to him when I do such things. As a wife, I feel that my actions are always helpful, but what I'm learning is that each time I make a gesture that allows me to "help" or "fix" the situation for him, it takes away more of his independence.

Over the years, I have found myself in seasons

of anger, loneliness, jealousy, resentment, worry, avoidance, extreme sadness, and overwhelming happiness. With each new challenge that presents, I may fail in my moment of weakness, but over time, I am able to look back and reflect on how the situation forced me to grow and change in positive ways.

Those days when I feel like I just can't do this anymore, I am blessed with little reminders in the form of friends, strangers, and coworkers to show that I am not alone. My current work as a social worker for children with special health care needs allows me to deeply understand the challenges and feelings of loneliness that families face on this journey. My position has been bittersweet. It often brings feelings of helplessness and inadequacy when I realize that I am struggling in similar ways as those I have been blessed with the opportunity to assist.

The journey has been long and hard for our

family, but especially for Bryan. Simple routine tasks to one person may be a much larger task for him on any given day. Each day I wake up with a choice in how I want my day to go.

I must continually remind myself that I have the power to choose how to focus my thoughts which will ultimately determine my mood for that day. Many days are met with mental, emotional, and physical exhaustion. But despite the overwhelming challenges, there are equally as many life-changing, eye-opening moments for our family. The quote that we have in our home says, "We may not have it all together, but together we have it all."

Despite the challenges, we have been blessed in a multitude of other ways. Bryan and I were happily married on March 17, 2007. Shortly after on July 9, 2007, we welcomed our son Christian. We again defied odds by becoming parents a second time and welcoming our daughter, Bryleigh, on December 7, 2009. These beautiful moments are memories I choose to focus on when the hard days come.

Despite all the possible outcomes, Bryan's overall health has remained fairly stable. While he is considered to be visually impaired, he does have sufficient vision to drive. Bryan struggles with focus, fatigue, frequent headaches, concentration, and memory loss. Compared to the alternative, he has been blessed with the best outcome.

When I picture our future, I see a 1,000 piece jigsaw puzzle that requires us to put it together piece by piece. Sometimes we try a piece that we are certain should fit tightly in a specific spot, but it just doesn't seem to fit. That does not stop us from still trying to force it a bit. This forced piece might fit for a short time, but when we attempt to attach the adjoining pieces, we quickly learn that we are assembling life's puzzle incorrectly. So, we backtrack and attempt to piece it together differently.

OUR LIFE PUZZLE

This puzzle can be pieced together, but the process might take a very long time. Some misplaced pieces. Some disassembly required. Not to mention an abundance of patience, dedication and commitment. We may even find a piece under the couch when we least expect it! Our life puzzle is not even partially complete. Like our daughter, we have taken a few breaks when we become overwhelmed with the magnitude of the puzzle. We always seem to find our way back to working hard to finish the puzzle.

I don't know what the future holds for our life puzzle, but I can guarantee that it will come with more trials and tribulations. When that life puzzle is close to completion, I know we will be filled with excitement at all we have accomplished.

—*Kallie Keith ©2020*

"Each new day is a blessing."

REFLECTIONS OF A CAREGIVER

In 1983, I met my husband, Paul, in Allentown, Pennsylvania, at a neighborhood pool. He was with his son. I was there with my friend, Miriam, who died of Alzheimer's this past March. Attracted to each other, we got to chatting.

A couple of weeks later, Miriam and I were out dancing on a Wednesday evening when we encountered Paul with his boss. They were both dressed in suits. I recognized him right away, but it took him a little while to recognize me. Finally, he said, "Is that you, Chris?"

We were married in 1988, a second marriage for both us. I never expected Alzheimer's would invade my husband's mind even though I knew his mother died of the disease, and it had plagued her sisters too. I had hoped retirement would bring perhaps a Viking Cruise down the Rhine, or a tour of Ireland, or Great Britain, or perhaps Tuscany with my vibrant and loving husband. But that will probably never happen.

Throughout 2019, I noticed changes in my husband's memory. I prodded him for months until he finally agreed to an appointment with his family doctor.

His primary doctor gave him a short memory test and ordered an MRI of his brain that did reveal some ischemic changes to the small blood vessels. His doctor said this was not unusual in older folks and referred Paul to a neurologist.

After enduring memory and cognitive tests, he was diagnosed with "mild cognitive impairment" which may or may not progress to Alzheimer's. He was given Donepezil (generic Aricept) and an antidepressant and told to come back in a year.

Fast forward to 2020. We went back for the same

tests. I was sitting next to him, and it was painful to hear him struggle to remember five words and repeat them at different times, draw a clock, count backward from 100 by three, name as many words that begin with an "f" in a minute as possible, and to remember that animal's name is a camel.

The nurse practitioner prescribed Memantine (generic Namenda) in addition to Donepezil, hoping to stop the progression of this horrible disease. At this appointment, she also recommended a driving evaluation because she feared if he were in an accident and it was revealed he had dementia, we could have serious liability problems. Although not happy about it, he voluntarily gave up driving until the evaluation. I was not surprised when the result of the evaluation was he should not drive anymore.

After the appointment, the nurse practitioner called and told me there was a significant decline in executive functions from last year. I pressed for a diagnosis. I was told Paul had moderate to severe Alzheimer's Disease mixed with vascular dementia. She came to this conclusion from the imaging tests and the cognitive tests. She requested that I tell Paul the news.

Reluctantly, on a beautiful night at our family cottage, I told Paul, but did not mention the severity of the diagnosis. He appeared to either not understand the diagnosis or to ignore it. Who wants to hear they have Alzheimer's Disease? I will never bring it up again unless he asks.

In his professional life, Paul was an accountant. Now, he cannot balance a checkbook. He readily gave the bill paying duties to me. Directions perplex him.

Personality changes continue to come. Never an angry person, he now becomes angry due to the frustration he encounters every day when he cannot find something or cannot express what he is feeling.

REFLECTIONS OF A CAREGIVER

For him, communicating effectively is practically impossible. When he is unable to find the right word, he will say "the thing." He is starting not to remember names of people he has not seen in a while, including his son's wife and their daughter. Although, I think if he saw them, he would know them.

His attention span is limited. Technology confounds him. The calendar confuses him. Every Sunday, I type up a schedule of what we are doing for that week. I cross out the days of the month on the calendar in the kitchen, so he can figure out what day of the week it is. Sometimes, I wonder if he looks at it.

His blood type is O negative, which is highly prized by the blood centers. After a few months of not giving blood, he made an appointment. I waited in the car for him. He arrived back in 10 minutes, clearly upset, because he was not allowed to donate blood. He was not able to give me a clear answer. It was something about his medications. I later learned he was rejected because they felt he could not understand the questions.

Paul keeps a list of his medications in his wallet. I think when he showed them the list, and they saw the dementia meds, it raised a red flag. Rejected, he was angry, humiliated, and embarrassed. It broke my heart. As my sister pointed out, "Paul was just trying to do good."

When we got home, I found him crying in the laundry room. He said he was stupid. I told him he was not stupid. It was the disease. I do not know if that comforted him or not.

Caring for a loved one with dementia is a very lonely and stressful experience. Although family and friends try to help as much as they can, they have their own lives to live. Unless they live the experience themselves, I think it is difficult for them to understand how lonely it really is.

To be an effective caregiver, I know I need to

take care of myself. I pray for patience every night. I pray to not get angry when he asks the same question repeatedly.

A person afflicted with Alzheimer's is always right. It does no good to argue with him, even if I am frustrated. He is unsure of himself, so all decision making is left to me. He is very dependent on me as that makes him feel safe. At times, that can be very constricting, such as when I am trying to have a private conversation with someone, or wanting to go to the store by myself to have some private time. My job is to be an advocate for my husband, which is a privilege. However, fear of the future is a reality. Will my husband eventually have to be in a nursing home? Will we have to sell our house? I worry about our finances. Right now, he is probably in stage three or four of the disease. How long will that last? Alzheimer's can span 8 to 20 years.

Sometimes, when Paul is having a bad day,

I look into his eyes and can see what it will be like when the light of recognition is gone. It is frightening to see the person you love slowly disappearing.

Right now, he takes care of himself, walks our dog, mows the lawn, and does household tasks. He took good care of me when I had my knee replaced in 2019. Sometimes he dresses colorfully. One day, he had on five t-shirts. When his siblings call, he always tells them he is doing fine.

For the most part, he is a cheerful and optimistic person—at least that is what he projects. His mother used to tell me he was the "helpful son." She had five sons. Paul always liked helping others. Even living with dementia, he still does. As one of my nieces said, "Uncle Paul has a heart of gold."

He is a very social person, much more than I am. With COVID-19 putting a stop to the Memory Cafés has been hard. Both of us especially liked going to the cafés at the Mosquito Hill Nature

Center because the talks were interesting and afterwards we could hike on the trails.

After thinking about events that transpired prior to 2019, I am sure Alzheimer's had been present for a few years. His primary doctor once told Paul he will never get better. Either the disease will progress on an even plane, or the plane would abruptly drop precipitously.

What do I miss? I miss a good conversation with him. I miss sleeping well consistently. I miss ballroom dancing lessons. I miss not worrying. I miss my husband as he was before the disease came.

Alzheimer's is a cruel and insidious disease. It robs its victim of his or her dignity and all that is precious to an individual. I will hope the current plane stays steady, but I don't think it will. I am grateful for our past together and will consider each new day a blessing.

—*Chris Calhoun* ©2020

"I choose to stay."

THE BEST AND THE WORST

There are two sides to being a family caregiver. There are the precious moments of joy and feelings of accomplishment and then there are the challenging moments that try to erase all those wonderful moments.

After 10 years of caring for my husband, I have come to realize that I have more control over the challenging situations than I initially thought. My attitude is everything. I cannot control his reaction, but I can control mine. I know this is not a new revelation, but it took me some time to come to this realization. Wasted time full of anger and resentment.

In the heat of the moment, it is so easy to get wrapped up in negative words and actions. Never argue with a person who has a cognitive disease is the #1 and most important rule that you learn. No matter how right you know you are and how wrong you know they are. Don't argue as you will never win. Save your energy for something more important. I know it is hard and it took lots of practice for me to get to this point.

Because of their disease, they truly believe what they are saying is right and they will seldom give in. Does it matter if they say they never watched a certain movie and yet you know they just watched it yesterday? Is it worth the effort it will have on your relationship with them? Nothing you can say or do is going to change what they believe, so save yourself some stress and agree. Later, you can scream in a pillow if you need to.

I have been told I need to learn to live in his world as he is not capable of living in mine. I admit there are times that I wonder which world I am in myself. Some days, I repeatedly have to

THE BEST AND THE WORST

agree that his mother is in a nursing home when I know she passed away five years ago. Having this conversation countless times, I feel I have even convinced myself that his mother is in a nursing home. I say that as a tongue in cheek statement.

My precious moments of joy are those rare glimpses that allow me to see my husband before this cognitive disease took him to another world. That gleam in his eye when he looks at me. His tender smile of affection. When he gently squeezes my hand. All these small interactions make me feel that the man I know and married is still in that body. He just has trouble expressing himself like he so lovingly used to.

I am committed to stay in this relationship for better or for worse.

—Choosing to Stay

*" Your intentions may
be well received."*

THE OTHER TALK

When you hear the words "The Talk," your first thought probably goes to when you had "The Talk" with your adolescent children. My children are grown and on their own. Now I am finding myself having "The Other Talk" with my parents.

Should they be driving? Should I take over their finances? Should they be living alone? Should they be living at home? Tons of questions with difficult answers.

I was dreading having to have "The Other Talk" with my parents. When I finally got up the nerve, I was surprised that they seemed relieved that I brought up the subject. In their mind, they thought they were doing a pretty good job of hiding the fact that they needed help. Yet they welcomed the intervention I was offering. What a load off my shoulders that was!

I have heard from others that "The Other Talk" is a most uncomfortable and difficult conversation to have with your parents. Once I started the conversation, everything just started to fall into place. I learned they had already started to check into places on their own. They admitted they have noticed changes themselves for awhile. They just wanted to be ready and to have a say in where they might move to next. I shared that I had been researching and even visiting facilities for them as well. I was pleased to see, based on our lists, that we agreed on a few places that would be a good fit.

Although they had noticed changes and were in agreement that they needed more care, neither one of them had taken the next step to talk to any doctors. That part of "The Other Talk" was a bit more difficult. When I explained testing was necessary for a move to take place, they finally agreed.

It was excruciating for me to be in the room with each of my parents separately to witness how difficult it was for them to answer some of the doctor's cognitive questions. Who is the president? What time of year is it? Can you draw a clock that shows 9:25? And the one test I am sure I would not possibly pass myself—"Remember these random words to repeat later." Yes, this short exam led to more testing for both my parents.

The test results were conclusive. Both parents had cognitive issues. The doctor recommended that I look for assisted living housing for them for now unless I had plans of moving in with them or they with me.

I love both my parents dearly, but with my career and my family, I felt I would not be doing justice to them. To prevent any resentment on my part or theirs, we came to a mutual agreement that an assisted living facility was a great decision. It would give them the watchful eyes that they needed 24/7 as well as some privacy and independence that they wanted to retain.

I felt the best solution would be to select a facility that offered various living options to allow my parents to receive additional care as they needed it without actually moving to another facility. The move happened about six months later and the transition could not have gone smoother. The fact that my parents were willing and ready to move made a world of difference.

As difficult as it feels, I would suggest having "The Other Talk" sooner than later with your parents. Maybe, like my parents, they are waiting for you to bring it up first. If not, at least you have broken the ice and you can talk with them about what they may have in mind for the future.

—Mary ©2020

"Have 'The Other Talk'
sooner than later."

A NOT SO LONELY JOURNEY

"What will the future bring?"

THE PERFECT LIFE

I always thought I was blessed with the perfect life. We were not rich, but we had all the basic needs. We never experienced what it is like to not have enough food. Sure, there were times when funds were short, but we always managed.

I had a hard-working, handsome husband who loved me, our definition of a dream home, and successful children. We have a son and a daughter which I have often heard referred to as the "million dollar family." As they say, life was good.

We were looking forward to fulfilling our early retirement dreams. We were about six months away from retiring when everything changed. Things were probably changing gradually for some time, but none of us realized what was happening.

Suddenly, our life became doctor appointments, testing, and an array of medications as the doctors tried to figure out what was going on with this 55 year old male. It felt like our life changed overnight. I was now the one who was, and probably would be, making all the decisions from this point forward.

This well-mannered man had now become verbally abusive, rude, outspoken, and frankly, just quite difficult. Many times it felt impossible to even take him anywhere for fear of what he may say or do. He would even scream obscenities at the neighbors. Thankfully, our neighbors were extremely understanding. As you can imagine, I spent a lot of time apologizing.

I often wondered if the array of medications were causing more issues than they were helping. The medication Aricept was used only two nights as it caused him to have terrible nightmares. Needless to say, neither of us got any sleep those two nights.

Yes, this disease called dementia, is slowly taking

him. Some days, I feel I see improvement, but then reality sets in. I often wonder what is it that makes some days better than others? Did he sleep better? Was it something he ate or didn't eat? I wish I knew the answers. There have been no med changes other than adding a mild anxiety medication which I feel helps to keep his temperament at a more even keel.

What is in store for us for the future? Only time will tell. From what I research, there is a strong possibility there will be a very distinctive change that will feel like it happened almost overnight. Or so it may seem. That may be when I will have to make the decision whether I can still care for him at home.

In the meantime, I am grateful for the memories of so many years of joy. Life changes, but memories do not. I still feel blessed in many ways, in spite of being my husband's caregiver.

—*Still Blessed*

"Find the right medical team."

THE RIGHT DOCTOR

I cannot say enough about the importance of finding the right doctor. How is that done? For us, it was trial and error. It was not easy.

At first, I depended on referrals from our family physician, family members, and friends. What they felt was a good fit for them, I often found was not a good fit for us.

I have read there are more than 400 types of dementia with the most common types being Alzheimer's and vascular dementia. The doctors are not quite sure what type my husband has so for now they just call it "not otherwise specified" or NOS. From what I understand, the medications and treatments prescribed vary depending on which type of dementia the patient has.

All this is a new road for us. I research what I can on my own. He sees specialists, but I still feel they do not fully understand dementia themselves. Most times, I still feel I understand more about dementia than they do because I am a caregiver for my husband. Yet I am not the one who is actually living with the disease itself. It appears with more than 400 types that are similar, it is difficult for even doctors to narrow it down. The mystery of the human mind is as amazing as it is complicated.

For us, the right doctor is someone willing to spend the necessary time to listen to my husband as well as myself. Actively listening and respecting what we both say. We had a few experiences where doctors seemed more worried about getting their "quota" in for the day than even taking time to make eye contact with us.

For now, we feel confident in his doctors. It was a long road to get there. I realize the day will come when they too will retire and we will again

THE RIGHT DOCTOR

be searching for the right doctor. For now, it feels good to have someone advocating for me as well as for my husband.

My advice? Do not give up and do not settle for a medical team that you and your loved one do not feel comfortable with. The search is worth the rewards it will reap.

—*Beth ©2020*

" *Caregiving is a badge of honor.*"

TREATED DIFFERENTLY

Since my husband, Steve, was diagnosed with Alzheimer's disease, it has been quite noticeable to me that family and friends act differently towards him. Before the diagnosis, they would call, visit, invite him to go golfing or to lunch. What a difference a day, or a diagnosis, can make. It was as if everyone, or perhaps just us, had fallen off a cliff and landed on a deserted island.

I suspect they did not know how to handle the news any better than I did. I needed my family and friends around me the most while I was dealing with the shock of the diagnosis. Perhaps they, too, were dealing with their own grief and really didn't know what to say?

Sure, I was probably in denial and deep down I

probably expected the diagnosis. My mind wanted to hear the words, "this prescription should take care of it in a couple of days."

Even more unexpected was how people were now treating ME. Not only family and friends, but co-workers and even managers at work.

I had always proven myself to be an outstanding employee and had worked hard to reach my status at work. At first, I was selective about who I shared the news about Steve with as I was still trying to process it myself.

Much to my surprise, as the "news" got out, I felt shunned. Was it my imagination? Even their good mornings seemed to have a sad pity tone. Where did their perky cheerfulness go?

One day, it came to my attention that a meeting I would normally have attended, was held without my receiving the usual invite. This was not a regularly scheduled meeting, but still it was a meeting that I would normally have been a part of.

I apologized to my manager for missing the meeting and explained to her that I had no record of receiving a notice to attend. She replied that she thought I had enough on my plate with Steve and didn't want to put more on my plate. My heart sank. Just because my husband has a cognitive disease, she thought I could no longer do my job? Did she think Alzheimer's is contagious?

In all honesty, I was speechless. That was not the response I expected from my manager and long time friend. She made the decision for me not to attend. I think it may have hurt even more because we had become close friends over the years.

She confirmed there were no complaints with my work. She just felt I should start carrying a lighter load when I was at work. I had worked so hard for years to earn the respect of my managers and co-workers, but now I had what appeared to me to be their pity.

It felt like I just slid to the bottom of the ladder

that I thought I was climbing. The ladder I worked so hard to climb over the past 12 years. My career was over – at least with this long-time employer. It was obvious, I would no longer be promotable in their eyes. At that moment, although I did not resign, I decided it was time to start over somewhere else. After all, it felt like I was starting over by having to prove that I can still handle my career along with my caregiving responsibilities at home.

With my education and experience, I was able to quickly land another position with better pay and better benefits. Funny how life pushed me into a better situation. However, I am still hurt by the experience, including the fact they did not try to talk me out of leaving. Hmm.

Ten years later, I am now retired. In looking back, I wonder why was I treated differently than a parent who had a young child at home or a parent of a child with a disability. Personally, I do not see the difference. There are adult day care facilities as well

TREATED DIFFERENTLY

as in-home care services. What is the difference?

I am pleased to see employers wanting to be educated on dementia as well as the caregiving aspects so they can understand that a person can be both a stellar employee and a stellar caregiver. In my opinion, the attitude towards dementia from the general public has changed drastically in the past 10 years. I feel being a family caregiver is a badge of honor. There is nothing to be ashamed of, nor should I need to hide the fact that I am a family caregiver for my spouse. By the way, I love "my new job" of caring for Steve.

—Aleda ©2020

"Will I survive?"

TWO STRANGERS IN THE HOUSE

I'm tired. I am physically tired and emotionally spent.

When this "journey" started over five years ago, I didn't think it would take this much of a toll on me. I made a promise to myself and a commitment to my husband, to not take him out of the home he worked so hard to build and the property we both love. But, this new job is wearing me down.

Accepting this life change was a slow, gradual process. Then one day, everything was crystal clear that the old life we shared was gone. There is a "stranger" in the house and I am in charge of taking care of him.

He looks the same, but that's just his outward appearance. He is morphing into someone new and someone I do not care for at times. Someone who is demanding, demeaning, unreasonable, mean, sometimes abusive, accusatory, suspicious and stubborn.

Showering is a battlefield. I've tried coaxing, begging, cajoling, pleading, bargaining. Hoping for that window of opportunity when he will cooperate. I have even let him go in the shower with his clothes on and then slowly remove his wet clothing. He was always neat in his appearance. Now I look at food stained clothes, sticky hair, and dirty fingernails.

How long can I hang on? What if this goes on for another 5 or 10 years? Will I survive? I don't think so.

The other "stranger" in the house is me. I, too, have become a stranger, someone I don't recognize. Someone who is seething on the inside, angry, resentful, impatient, withdrawn, unhappy, and scared.

I want to lash out at friends or avoid them completely. I certainly don't want to share in any of their good news or happiness. I'm resentful that I can't spend time with our grandchildren. My anger and resentment is making me a bitter person. Someone that I don't care for. Amazing how anger can overpower all other emotions such as love, compassion, kindness, and empathy.

I have found that if I adjust and lower my expectations that it becomes easier to deal with the disappointments. Sometimes I will plan a surprise outing, not far, just a drive and maybe a stop at a favorite shop to browse or get an ice cream cone. Preparing for something like this can become a war of wills when he refuses to put socks and shoes on or leave his chair. Plans canceled!

I feel diminished. My daily tasks seem bigger and I feel smaller. When do I throw in the towel? I get so angry at him and feel so bad for him at the same time.

Being kind to both "strangers" is hard some days. I now understand what collateral damage means. I have been taken down by this horrible disease as have our daughters and their families, relatives, and friends.

Our grandchildren have missed getting to know an interesting grandfather who had endless adventure stories to tell about his work around the world as a geologist. His excitement in teaching science. His love of nature.

Hopefully one day I'll be able to recreate those adventures for them in writing and pictures so his memory will not be that of the strange man sitting in his chair yelling at the TV.

The "long goodbye" is an understatement!

—*Rose ©2020*

TWO STRANGERS IN THE HOUSE

"Keeping memories alive."

A NOT SO LONELY JOURNEY

"Don't set expectations."

WHAT I WISH I HAD KNOWN

The disease is going to continue to progress. You can't buck it, make it better, or make it go away.

You have to set aside your natural instinct of reacting, and your emotions.

Rubbing her back, giving her hugs, and physical contact can be very calming.

Don't expect her to learn. She does not have that ability anymore and will repeat the same mistakes day after day.

Don't expect empathy for your aches and pains. She only occasionally has that ability.

Don't expect efficiency. You'll be disappointed. In fact, don't have expectations. You'll be frustrated.

Say "I'm sorry" even when you don't know what you're sorry for.

Don't expect her to say "I'm sorry."

Don't expect her to hurry. She'll move even slower.

Plan ahead. Allow at least an extra half hour to make any appointment.

When you ask her to do something and she is resistant, let it lie. She may come around to doing it later on her own.

If she doesn't want to do something, it does no good to argue with her or to try to convince her. It only makes matters worse.

Agree, agree, agree.

—*John Weyers ©2020*

WHAT I WISH I HAD KNOWN

"It does no good to argue."

A NOT SO LONELY JOURNEY

"Angels on Earth."

WHAT IS A CAREGIVER?

Loving. Patient. Kind. Calming. Advocate. Nurse. Cook. Housekeeper. Accountant. CEO. Chauffeur. Personal Shopper. Teacher. Repairperson. Activity Director. Friend. Mother. Sister. Spouse. Aunt. Grandmother. Employee. Manager. All that and so much more. Sounds like a super woman, doesn't it? At times, it feels like it. At the end of the day, I wonder how I accomplished so much and on some days so little.

I feel I am a single mother to a spouse who is two years old. A spouse who needs me to manage his temper tantrums at home and in public. He has lost all sense of how to act appropriately as an adult. I understand this is part of the disease, but it is difficult to comprehend sometimes.

One of my biggest frustrations is I see a grown man who is not capable of taking any of the daily chores off my shoulders. Instead, I find myself tripping over and picking up his shoes which he will leave wherever he feels the need to take them off. He insists on putting his shoes on when he gets dressed. If he gets dressed. Most nights, he insists on sleeping in his clothes. It's a battle I rarely win.

I clean up messes in the bathroom and quite frankly, I am cleaning up after him 24/7. He does nap often which gives me time to catch up. Just as I think I might have a few moments for myself, he is up from his nap and the cycle begins again.

There are days that I wonder if his actions are to spite me? With a grin, he will watch me clean up his messes. I have to remind myself, again and again, it's the disease affecting his cognitive abilities in spite of what my eyes tells me.

Some days are more difficult than others, but I continue to choose to care for my husband. I made

WHAT IS A CAREGIVER

a vow "in sickness and in health" 40 years ago. I intend to keep that vow as long as I am physically and mentally able.

I have heard it said that caregivers are angels on earth. I do not feel I deserve to be put into that category most days, but I do like the thought of it.

—*Sally* ©2020

"I have no regrets."

WHERE DID THE LAUGHTER GO?

I used to wonder where the fun went that used to be a big part of our lives. Our life was full of smiles and laughter. We had a full social life with very few open dates on our calendar.

After we received Wayne's diagnosis, everything became grim and dark. The laughter and smiles disappeared. We barely even talked that week. I am sure we were both digesting the information in our own way and scared what the future would hold.

I knew the silence had to be broken, so I approached Wayne. "What were his first thoughts? What would be our next step? What can I do to help?" It was still hard for him to share, but with prodding Wayne opened up.

It never occurred to me to leave, so I was a bit surprised when Wayne told me his first thoughts were that I would leave him. Wayne went on to encourage me to leave as he did not want to become a burden causing me to resent him. His statements left me somewhat wondering if he would have chosen to leave me if the situation were reversed.

It was a much needed long, powerful, and emotional discussion, but I eventually convinced Wayne that I wanted to stay and I assured him I would not resent him. That was then and this is now.

I admit that I had no clue how much caring for Wayne was going to change our relationship or how difficult it would become. I have no regrets, but I certainly was not prepared for what the future would bring.

Each day, I do my best trying to bring joy back into our lives. I can sense that looking at old pictures, other than our wedding day, makes

WHERE DID THE LAUGHTER GO

Wayne sad. I share silly jokes with Wayne that I find and look for sitcoms and comedy genre movies to watch together. Occasionally, I make funny faces which usually gets a giggle or a smile from Wayne. Perhaps my only regret is that we did not have children. I often think what joy grandchildren would bring to us now. It's not easy, but I feel each day is what I make of it.

—Sue ©2020

*"Thank you for this
opportunity to be part of
your journey!"*

THANK YOU

We are honored and humbled to be trusted with compiling the sharing of these thoughts and journeys to make this book possible. All credit goes to the amazing caregivers who were eager to share to support other family caregivers.

This collection is shared in the caregivers' own words. Through this sharing, it is the hope that other caregivers will find comfort and that family members, friends, co-workers, and employers will come to better understand the journey of dementia caregivers.

We are confident that as a caregiver, family member, friend, co-worker, or employer, you will find valuable information shared in this book.

Which sharing touched you the most? Which

are your favorites? We would like to hear from you. Contact us at FamilyCaregiversRock@outlook.com or through the website FamilyCaregiversRock.org.

Although the journey seems lonely at times, caregivers are truly never really alone as shared by these amazing family caregivers.

CC Thompson and Walter Zerrenner

AFTERWORD

Whether you are a family caregiver, family member, friend, co-worker, employer, or medical provider, it is our hope you were able to take away something from what these amazing family caregivers have shared.

A NOT SO LONELY JOURNEY

"You are not alone."

ABOUT

CC THOMPSON became a family caregiver at the age of 17. In 2012, CC made the decision to retire early to be the primary caregiver for a family member.

In talking with other family caregivers in the fall of 2017, the idea came about to publish a collection of caregiving journeys to support family caregivers on their journey. The book, *A Lonely Journey*, was published in March 2018.

In recognition of CC's support of family caregivers through her work on the book, CC received the honor of being named a 2018 Family Caregiver of the Year at the National Caregiving Conference in Chicago.

In November of 2018, again in conversation with other family caregivers, the idea came about to form a nonprofit called Family Caregivers Rock that would grant wishes to family caregivers. CC became a founding member and continues to serve on the volunteer board today. The nonprofit's mission has since expanded to "Supporting the health and wellness of Wisconsin family caregivers through community projects, events, and granting wishes to family caregivers."

In 2019, several local and national magazines published articles about CC's support of family caregivers through her work on the first book as well as the nonprofit.

In 2020, CC was again honored for her support of family caregivers and was presented with a Northeast Wisconsin Remarkable Women award.

With the support of the Aline Zerrenner Dementia Friendly Fund, CC and Walt Zerrenner began working on the second book, "A Not So Lonely Journey," in June 2020.

CC was born and raised in Northeast Wisconsin. She has been married to her high school sweetheart for 44 years. They have been blessed with a son and his wife, a daughter, a granddaughter and three grandsons.

WALTER ZERRENNER has cared for his wife Aline since 2007, when she was first diagnosed with Mild Cognitive Impairment (MCI). Today, Aline has advanced Alzheimer's and has resided in memory care since December 2014.

Walt's career was in the field of information technology beginning in 1963 following his honorable discharge from the Marine Corps. The last 25 years before his retirement, he was a Senior VP for a large healthcare system responsible for the information technology divisions.

He and Aline married in 1965, and have two children and five grandchildren. Walt currently serves on three nonprofit boards and facilitates three support groups for men caring for their wives who are living with dementia.

In 2017, Walt was named the Alzheimer's

ABOUT

Association Family Caregiver of the Year and received senatorial recognition from a U.S. Senator for his work as a caregiver.

In 2020, Walt received the Paul and Elaine Groth Mentoring Award which was sponsored by the Mielke Family Foundation.

Direct all medical and legal questions to your medical and legal professionals.

DISCLAIMER

These thoughts and journeys are written and shared by family caregivers in their own words, not by medical or legal professionals.

Any information shared in this book is not intended to be, nor should it be, interpreted as medical or legal advice.

Medical and legal questions or concerns should be directed to your medical and legal professionals.

*"May you find comfort and
support on your journey."*